SADHANA GUIDELINES

FOR KUNDALINI YOGA DAILY PRACTICE

Based on the Teachings of Yogi Bhajan

ACKNOWLEDGEMENTS

Guidelines to a Successful Sadhana would never have been possible without our Teacher, Yogi Bhajan (Siri Singh Sahib Bhai Sahib Harbhajan Singh Khalsa Yogiji). From cover to cover, these are the teachings he has given us. Our gratitude to him is infinite.

M.S.S. Gurucharan Singh Khalsa, Ph.D.
Kundalini Research Institute
Pomona, California
December, 1976

Published by
Kundalini Research Institute
P.O. Box 351149
Los Angeles, CA 90035

DEDICATION

This manual is dedicated to Yogi Bhajan (Siri Singh Sahib Bhai Sahib Harbhajan Singh Khalsa Yogiji) and to that golden chain of teachers and students extending from the Infinite Teacher, linking us all together through time and space as we are each, in turn, students to our teachers and teachers to our students.

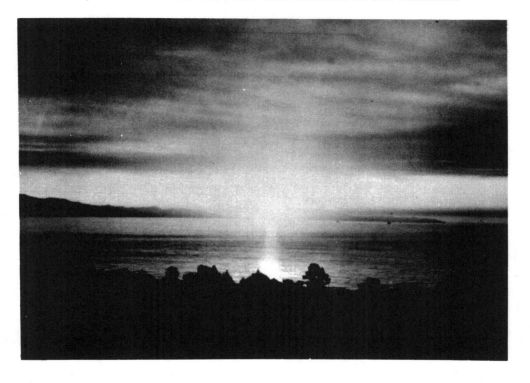

HUKAM

Say, what lies with a man to do or not?
Only the Lord causes to happen what He will.
If man had the power, he would seize everything to himself.
But he can do only what the Lord wants done.
Not knowing this, man dwells with illusion,
For if he knew, would he not save himself?
But deluded by doubt, he wanders in all directions,
And rushes forth to explore all the four continents.
When, however, out of His Mercy, God grants His love,
Man absorbs himself in the practice of the Name.

"Sadhana gives one a disciplined practice
to integrate the body, mind, and spirit."

Yogi Bhajan, PhD

TABLE OF CONTENTS
SADHANA GUIDELINES

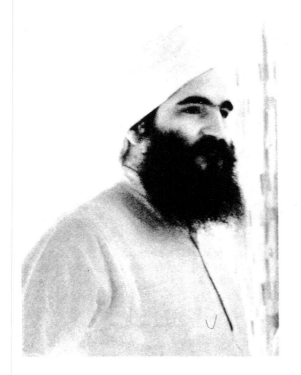

INTRODUCTION

By Mukhia Singh Sahib Gurucharan Singh Khalsa

This manual is designed for both the new and the experienced student. It focuses on the essential practice of Kundalini yoga: *sadhana*. Quite a bit of new material has been added since the first edition. A section on basics and several beginners sets are to aid the use of this manual in the many college courses now being tought. The three lectures by Siri Singh Sahib Bhai Sahib Harbhajan Singh Khalsa Yogiji were added to give a broader introduction to the nature of Kundalini yoga and meditation.

All of the thought, inspiration, and techniques for this manual have come to us from the Siri Singh Sahib. His openness and true humility in sharing the knowledge and secrets of the sages, the truths distilled from ages of human experience, is the keynote of the Aquarian Age. Any mistakes are those of this scribe, not of the teacher.

The Siri Singh Sahib spoke about sadhana at the Winter Solstice celebration in December, 1973, in Orlando, Florida. This excerpt from his informal talk summarizes the essence and spirit of all the pages to follow. If this statement is taken to heart and put into practice, all other questions will be answered.

A sadhu is a being who has disciplined himself. Sadhana is the technique to discipline yourself. Those who create separation in sadhana have not yet crossed the barriers of their mind and ego. I will show you by example. I don't know how you can be so idiotic to say someone who is doing a sadhana can create terrible problems when actually he is blessed.

Once we invited a teacher to Guru Ram Das Ashram and he chose to speak on Kundalini yoga. He told me to come and sit by his side. I said, 'Nothing doing. You are my guest and at any one time, one teacher speaks.' So I made him sit there and I sat in the area where the students sit. We listened to 45 minutes of his speech against Kundalini yoga, very calmly and very quietly, and it didn't bother us. In the end he asked me to give a closing remark. I got up and said, 'God bless you. You have given us a chance to think how faithful we are.' And that's it.

A sadhana is a sadhana. In sadhana, if *Jap Ji* is read, let everybody read it. Let everybody sing with it, let everybody glorify himself. Or if there is a Grace of God course, where the ladies are participating and they just want to participate separately, let the men go into a silent prayer. Say, 'God, really make them a grace of God so that they will get off our backs!' Do you see what I mean? We always can help each other so there is no problem. But we have a habit of doubting everything to the extent that we become a living doubt! Doubt, doubt, doubt, everything doubt.

I feel that in the morning, when you go for sadhana, you are going to be sadhus. What does it matter if somebody just gets up to say, 'Hmmm Hmmm?' That person is still doing it! He is doing *something*; he is not sleeping. It is far better than a person who is snoring. Do you understand? Sadhana is a willful effort to prove you are not lazy about your own infinity. When the sun rises early in the day, even idiots rise; but blessed are those who rise before the sun to prove that they are sons and daughters of the Almighty. Does it sound clear to you? At 3:30 p.m. you will probably get up. But those who have the guts will open up the gates of the heart at 3:30 a.m., they will love their Lord, they will communicate with their God and they will tell Him, 'Whether you belong to us or not, we belong to you.' That is all it's about.

It is a time and a process where people get up in the morning to chant the glory of the Lord, in this way or in that way, and then they clean their temple. This is how sadhana takes place at the Golden Temple in Amritsar, India. When we first go to the temple, we take away everything, clean the floors, then give the marble a bath with milk. We clean and polish every part of it, then redecorate it. Then at 3:00 a.m. the gates open and the sangat is allowed to come. The sangat chants there from 3:00 to 5:00 a.m. and then, in a golden palki sahib, the *Siri Guru Granth Sahib* is brought in. At 7:00 a.m. the hukam* is taken. Those who have gone to the Golden Temple know it.

In your own sadhana it is exactly the same way. Your body is the temple of God, and your soul is the divine Guru within. So you get up in the morning; you meditate; you chant the mantras; you do the exercises; you call on your spirit; you regulate the breath; and you get together in group consciousness because it helps each other. That is what morning sadhana and group consciousness is: It is a help to each other.

If I am trying to sleep, another is not sleeping. If in this whole group one person opens up to God just once, we all will be blessed in His openness. That is what matters. If one has walked into sadhana with heart and soul in a prayerful mind, we all will be benefited. That is the power of the group sadhana. All should participate. But you know, we still have something of the past in us. We bring up worries about who should lead: "Oh, that leader has brought a very good sadhana; that one has freaked out the sadhana." We go through this every day. The truth is that nobody freaks out the sadhana and nobody makes it beautiful; it is the Will of God which prevails through the soul. When you are a servant and act as a channel, it prevails through you; when you are clogged up and mugged up it doesn't come through. That's what it is.

somebody other than a Sikh (Sikh means a seeker of the truth), what can I say to him? If in the morning sadhana one cannot curtail the barriers and get to the oneness, I don't think there is any other time it can happen. One for all, because all is for one. That's the principle.

*The Sikh scripture contains teachings and songs of divine inspiration of both Sikh gurus and Hindu and Muslim saints and bards ranging from the 12th through the 17th centuries. A hukam is a verse chosen at random from the *Siri Guru Granth Sahib*, read each morning as the direction for the day.

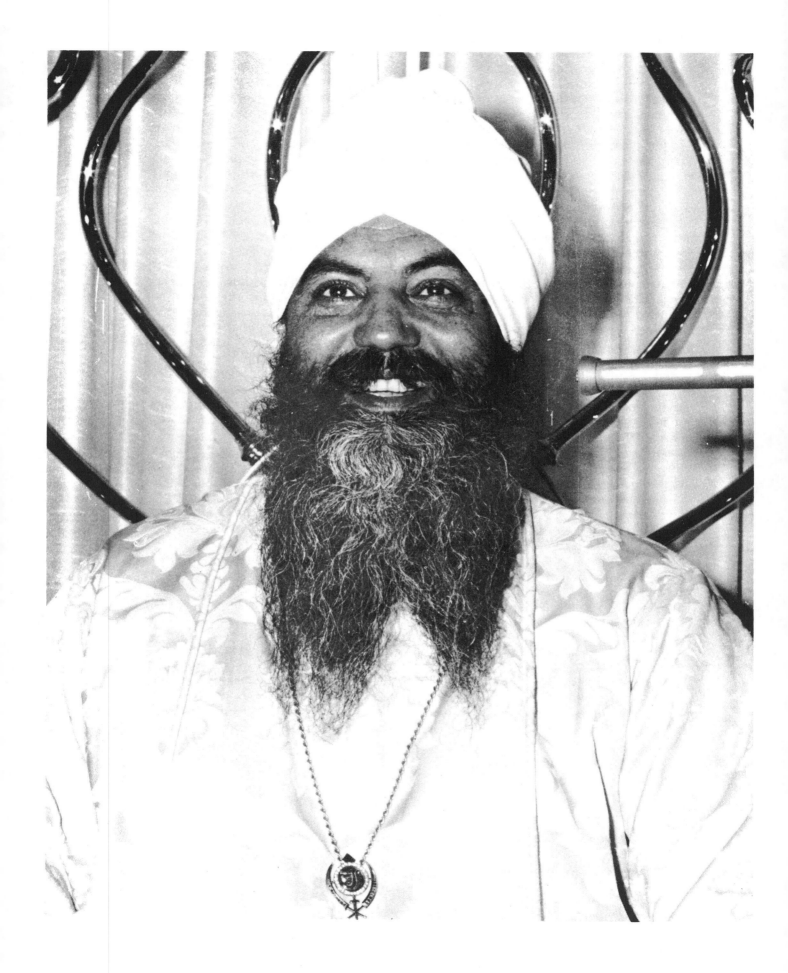

What Is Yoga?

An Adventure in Awareness

By Siri Singh Sahib Bhai Sahib

Harbhajan Singh Khalsa Yogiji

I have just completed a national tour today. On my tour I found that people do not have a basic understanding about yoga. Some people think yoga is a religion. Some people think it is for vitality and health. Some people think it is to promote their personality. In reality, this is all a misunderstanding. The word *yoga*, as we in the West understand it has come down from the biblical word, *yoke*. If you go to the original word in Sanskrit, it is *jugit*. The definition of a yogi is a person who has totally leaned on the supreme consciousness, which is God. *Yoga is the union of the individual's unit consciousness with the infinite consciousness.* That is all it means.

Classically, your potential self is infinite, whether you know it or you don't know it. The fact remains that every human mind belongs to infinity and to creativity. But in practical action, it is limited. So a technical know-how is required through which a man can expand his mental faculties in order to bring about the equilibrium to control his physical structure and experience his infinite self. That's all yoga means in very simple terms.

In this life of ours, yoga is greatly needed. Today the human being does not understand why he is a human being or what it means to be a human being. Talking about his infinity and knowing and experiencing infinity is a big deal. Remember that wisdom does not hold you. Wisdom only becomes knowledge when you experience it. Only the experience of that knowledge, *gyan*, can hold and support you. Just because you know or believe something to be true does not mean that you can act on it. But if you know truth and act on that path, and if you find bliss, success and fulfillment in yourself, then no power on earth can make you do wrong. Once you have seen the joy of that truth and have enjoyed that beauty you are okay. Some people misunderstand this. They say *knowing* the truth is alright. They say wisdom is good, but knowledge is not good. Wisdom becomes knowledge when it becomes your personal experience. And anything which can hold and support you is knowledge. A guru can give you wisdom but he cannot give you knowledge. And this is where we normally mess ourselves up. We think that so and so is a wise man. Learning from him, serving him, feeling good about him will make

everything alright. But no, it never works that way. He can give you the technical know-how but the knowledge is yours. His is the wisdom. So he has an essential part to play in this, but you are an equally essential part.

The first factor as a human being is to understand your vehicle, the physical or gross body. You have a very complicated inner machinery. It is not just the flesh and bone you can see. It's a very systematic system. It has glands, blood circulation, a breathing apparatus, heart-beat pulsation, a brain, and a total nervous system. All those systems combined over a structure of flesh and bone constitutes your physical system. It is a functional system. Whatever is a functional system needs cleaning, needs care, needs tuning. It also needs careful assessment of its capacity of activity, its potential to be extended, and its possibilities of longevity. All that has to be taken care of to start with.

If somebody wants to mess himself up all he has to do is overeat. After ten or fifteen days he'll be in the hospital. There's no problem. In New York I met a case. I said, "Why are you on welfare?" He said, "I can't hold myself together." It surprised me. His problem was that he overate. He would get sick and go to the hospital. After he got out they would ask him to take precautions and not do it again. But he would immediately overeat, get sick, and go back in. It was a total cycle.

The physical body is the basic temple in which you can deposit the treasure of happiness of life. You have to understand it. When you are young you can play mischief with the physical body. But in old age the body has you paying for the playing. You can never get out of it. So the body has to be scheduled. You have to calculate on a sliding scale. Suppose I must live a hundred years. Now, I have to plan for that. How should I carry this model 1929, or whatever model it is? From that year you want to live a hundred years. Now, if you buy a car in 1970 for a single driver, you can expect that with regular service, oil changes, etc. that it will get a certain mileage. But if you do not schedule it practically, after two years you will have to change the car. You are very happy to change a car because it gives you status in society, and a new car is good to drive all the time. But it doesn't work that way with the human body. You are not so fearless that after five or ten years you can say, "Alright, I can change the human body, I can get into another." You have not developed your individual consciousness to universal consciousness so that you can do it. There are people, there have been human beings, who have done it. It's not an unusual feature. But mostly people do not know how to do that. Therefore it is essential to make the best of what you have.

In this course, we will study the human body in the light of yoga therapy to make it understandable to you and show how you can make the best use of it. You must be able to keep it on the level of consciousness you choose so that it can serve you better and better without a lot of trouble. That's the maximum you can do.

A second factor in our human life is our mind. If the horizon of thought and understanding, tolerance and patience is limited, and if the mind is not so beautifully functional that it can see the unseen, and understand the consequences of actions, it is practically impossible to live a happy life. Because if you do not have a road map, you do not know where you are going. Then what are you doing? Just driving? That's what we do in life. I don't want to pull your leg tonight. I want you to feel very happy and good, but I have to give you a basic human assessment and overview.

What is the aim of your life? "Oh, everything is alright." What is alright? Nothing! Ask anybody. Everybody has twenty complaints about himself. Why? Where does the time go? Early in the morning, you go to the office and earn money. Saturday you have to pay your bills and buy the groceries. If there's a long weekend you have to take care of your taxes. Three hundred and sixty-five days go like this. Only leap year adds an extra day and that only comes after four years. We are that involved in life that we don't know any better. And when we do not know any better, how's the better going to come? We have passed our years with such speed that we do not know how we are maintained, except with God's blessing.

This functional structure of a human machine is so beautifully made by the Maker that it can recover from normal jerks and problems. It is a real and very rare mental shock that can damage your mental energy. When there is constant pressure and no relaxation, when there is no outlet or when there is constant boredom in life or a constant cavity in the capacity of mental life, it results in a shattered mind and the loss of happiness. Then you must get to a psychiatrist or a counselor or some yogi or do something. You have to depend on someone. Then every wise man will have to put a string in your nose and carry you through. But I don't believe in that. I believe every man represents God.

There are three basic letters in the word "God": G-O-D. These letters stand for the generating principle, the organizing principle, and the destroying principle. What we have done is taken the first letter from each of those three words and combined them together to make the word "God." God is not a guy standing on a seventh sky at the head of time watching you. It is the generating principle. It is infinity to infinity in relationship to the total creativity. Through its changing, everything happens. We have been brainwashed, but that has to be clearly understood.

We always say, "When I pray, God will come," What is prayer? Have you ever understood what a prayer is? You create a vibratory effect, it goes into the infinite creativity around your psyche, and the answer comes and is expressed in the energy of a job done. Then you say, "Well, prayer works." It is only your mind which has the power to concentrate and to work with that beauty.

Remember you have three aspects. You have the lower self, the gross or physical self; you have the central self, which is known as the existing self; and you have the higher self, which is a powerful, sophisticated and delicate self. So you can work on any level and you can go up and down, but you have to train yourself through your own experience. You can get knowledge from A, B, and C. It doesn't matter. If you can get wisdom from anybody, it is always a beautiful bounty. It is a special treat if you find some person who can stand by you and let you go through that experience. You are a God-conscious individual because you have the power of mental infinity.

I am talking in two languages now. In one word I am saying it scientifically, in the other I am relating in a mystic language. This way you can understand both. When you say, "I am a God-conscious person," it only means that you realize your mental capacity and ability. There is nothing more than that because everything you have is your mind. If somebody is beautiful or ugly to you, it is your mental evaluation. Somebody seems rich to you even though he doesn't give you a penny. He is rich to you because of *your* mental appraisal. You may imagine somebody is poor, even though the guy may have a million dollars sitting right under his seat. You call him poor because of your own mind. Actually, everything is your mental outlook. The problem with your mind is that as you think, so you are. How can man develop his mental faculty to perceive everything correctly? I would like to train you that way so that you may have a happy life around you.

The third factor as a human being is the soul, the spirit. As no lamp can burn without methylated spirit in it, so no life can exist without a relationship of spirit in it. Spirit has many meanings, tones and facets. If there is a central thread in it, all it is, is the general flow of the cosmic energy. In Catholicism we call it God, in yoga we call it cosmic energy. The meanings are exactly the same.

You have to understand your physical relationship with that infinite energy and how you can tune in for your own purposes, so that you can have a healthy, happy, holy, wholesome life, a fulfilled life, a beautiful life in which you can perceive in yourself the contentment of existence. You should be so contented that if you had to quit this planet you would just say, "Thank you." You have got to give thanks. And if the bad times are coming, just say, "Wonderful." Good days are coming, say, "Fine."

After all, what is life? It is a wave. The light must follow the night as night must follow the day. Sunshine must follow the clouds, clouds must follow the sunshine. But you feel you are really something special. You want sunshine all the time. If man is in the sun all the time the nose gets burned and the eyes can't see. No one can live in this world with sunshine all the time. Is there anyone willing to do that? No. This up and down is the beauty. Having happiness all the time is a very boring thing. You can't live that way. You have to have a little pull sometimes and just feel where you are and where you should be. That's why we call this life a vibration. What is a vibration, actually? Vibration is that which vibrates. And what is it? A path of vibration. Up and down! A wave. As a wave moves, so life moves. What do we want out of it? What do we desire? We desire a mind which is neutral, which understands the wave. You all know about surfing? When there are heavy tides people go surfing. They enjoy it. Other people go crazy. A mind which is developed, artistic, and self-controlled rides on those waves in life and enjoys it.

If a person with such a mind experiences a bad time, he can sit down and say, "Oh, God! Wonderful! What do you want? A bad time? So, what's it to me? I don't care." He communicates, he talks, he feels the fun. He's not upset. He knows after this night there will be a good warm day. He's going to have a lot of fun. So he preserves his energy. He keeps himself together. When the time comes that he can expand and enjoy, he comes out with all his energy to enjoy it all the way. That quality of mind has to be developed. It has to be trained; it has to be made and felt. The faculty and the capacity of the mind has to be geared into those grooves of action. If that is not possible, nothing is possible. This process is another important part of yoga.

Actually Kundalini yoga means awareness. Awareness is a finite relationship with infinity. That's what it means. This dormant energy is in you. This awareness is sleeping in you and you only experience your capacity to a limit. But when it can be extended to infinity you remain you, anyway. But in that state there is nothing lacking. This is what is called the basic human structure, the framework through which we have to function. Do you like it? Are you willing to agree to all this? I'm going to focus on this structure and its work. I do not know whether you will agree with me and I don't want you to agree with me. Remember one thing:

don't agree with me anywhere. If you have any point of disagreement, come out with it. I love argument, but I want another man to provoke it. I don't want to put a question in the mind of the people.

We all want to have good health. Many people feel we get sick because we do not know better. My personal feeling is very different. I don't believe that anybody wants to be unhealthy. But I also don't believe we do not go unhealthy. We do. We go and get sick sometimes.

There are two types of sicknesses: intentional and unintentional. Intentional sickness is when we know we are going to get sick but we still do it. I get into intentional sickness very often and I know that. Do you think a man of my awareness is an idiot since for 18 days I didn't get any sleep? I am not aware I'm going to get into trouble? From the day I put myself on the plane and started on tour until I returned today I didn't get the chance to sleep even though I tried. The schedule was automatic, the demand was heavy: from one meeting to another meeting, discussion after discussion, etc. We opened up our drug program with a press conference in Washington. After that everybody became curious. The news spread. Then people would not let us sleep. The subconscious mind did not allow us not to do sadhana. We also let anybody who wanted to talk to me have a chance. If somebody wants to know something we must share with him. You sometimes ask why I just don't share. But I can't do that. I thought we would have five days of rest in Canada. To my surprise they had a full schedule and I said, "Alright. WE will not go by any schedule. Anybody can come in." That was the only way to safeguard that all the services would be completed. I was aware that I was getting sick intentionally. The body can only go to a certain extent. You can ride a horse, and you can go on beating it. But it can only go a certain number of miles before it will start dropping. These are intentional sicknesses.

There are also unintentional sicknesses. For that I have a lot of compassion. We do not know how to eat, we do not know how to digest, we do not know how to live, we do not know how to take care of this body and we do not worry about whether our glands are functional or whether our nervous system if alright. We do not know to check if our cleaning is perfect or our rest and activity are balanced. That is unawareness. And that makes us sick. And that is where the main pain lies. This is especially true in this society today.

This morning I was talking on television. I told them that I had to catch a flight and I had to go. They said, "Well, you cannot leave that way. We definitely have to talk to you. Not all the people could come to that church to see you because the church had a limited space; it couldn't hold more than five hundred people. The people have forced us to have you come and answer certain questions on the television." I think T.V. is the best way to get into the living room without breaking into the house. Television is quite a procedure. You get into that box and you talk about anything you like.

When I went on that program they were having a discussion with a trained specialist, an expert, who does not believe in marriage. He feels marriage is going to be wiped out of the western countries. It is the most unrequired thing of the past. I asked him, "Then why are you talking about it?" He said, "I don't think it's essential." I said, "Well, your mother must have married your father. That's why you are discussing it with me today. Your existence is out of that action which should come out of the matrimonial relationship." And he said to me, "I want to ask a question." I said, "Well, go ahead. You are very anti-marriage, and I am very much for it. You are an outcome and a by-product of a marriage. Therefore, you cannot speak too heavily against it." We had twenty minutes of laughing and happiness. I enjoyed it and he enjoyed it.

Later on when the interview was over he said, "I am a great fool. I have made a total idiot of myself before all of Canada. (This was a coast-to-coast program.) What have I done to myself? I thought you were a simple yogi and that I would take you left and right." I said, "I am very simple. That's why I asked you very simple questions. You thought that by asking me two or three of the intellectual type questions you could just blow me up. But that is not true. You have to raise your mind to the capacity of my mind, and you will overcome it. If you don't have that mind, you are limited. You are just intellectually trying to argue left and right. But what is left and right about truth?"

To approach yoga in its totality, you have to know what living is. You have to know what a relationship is, what values this life can give you. If you know what you want then you can find it. Without any knowledge, are you just going to close your eyes and start walking? Where will you go? "I am going to the beach." You don't know. You may end up in the mountains. You have to keep yourself re-aimed. Your compass must tell you at what altitude, latitude and longitude you are going. It is a totally planned life because the "o" of the word, "God," G-O-D, means organization.

We often misunderstand or deny our basic nature in our social habits and communication. First of all, we are people of faith. Our first impulse and our greatest capacity is faith. Suppose we find a happy man. We know he is a good man and that he talks truthfully. We believe him. If he says something, we can act on it, and we can get happiness. Then we share it. But we do not relate this way. Instead of receptivity, we say, "Well, why are you happy? Convince me before I listen. I don't believe you." We always live on our insecurity. We cannot hide it. We cannot discuss anything with any other human being without first questioning his personality. "Who are you? What are you doing? How can you say that?" Why do we ask those questions? First of all, we do not know who we are.

Actually, we can go through life in two styles. We can act as if everybody were thieves until proven saints. Or we can act as if everybody were saints until proven thieves. Which style of life your mind has as a conception and an action depends on how strong a nervous system you have. People who live one style walk on every walk of life with an even attitude. If you ask them, "How are you doing?" They reply, "Oh, I am fine." If there are certain dangers they might encounter they say, "Oh, I don't care. No danger is going to bite me." People who live in the other style are completely different. If you tell them, "The road is clear. It has been checked. It is beautiful," they will say, "Oh, I don't believe it. I can't go. I can't walk further."

The basic insecurity in mental attitude and structure is often very elemental to a person's consciousness. I counseled a particular case in Washington, D.C. We discussed everything. There was a little marriage dispute, something normal. We cleaned it out. But the man said, "I understand that she has understood the mistake and when she understands, she never acts wrongly. But still, I can't believe her." She said with anger and frustration, "The thing that bugs me the most is that he always says he can't believe me!" When I went deeper into his personality I found that his not believing the woman came from his background of experienced knowledge that he got from the activity of his mother. It took me four hours to tell him, "Your mother was your mother, and this woman is your wife." He said, "That is my problem. I can't always believe it." So I said, "What are you up to? Don't you understand that she is your wife, not your mother? Why do you want to punish this lady because of your mother?" Then he told me that he had spent thousands of dollars going from one expert to another and still didn't know anything better. I said, "Alright. I'll tell you another way. Go and buy beads." So he bought the beads the next day. I said, "When you talk to this lady, catch your beads with a hand. Forget you are talking for a few seconds and remember that you are catching something." He said, "What does that do?" I said, "It will remind you that you are talking to your wife, not your mother. Simple. Whenever you talk to this lady who is your wife, put a hand on the beads and remember that you are not talking to your mother. You are talking to a wife. You married her. She's your life partner." He said, "Well, a woman is a woman." I said, "But with this woman you share a bed. With your mother you don't. You were a little child when you did that. So please be mature." I had to be practical and go very deep into his basic foundations of life in order to dig him out of his insecurity. Then he could start a new life by himself.

In every mental state of mind the subconscious plays a large role of which we are not aware. We all think we know "my past." There is no such thing as "my past." That past is only the experience you have in your subconscious mind and it does not let you move forward in your life. In Kundalini yoga, we fry this subconscious mind. We make a toast out of it and eat it. It is one of the best dishes we make. We have a technical know-how to approach this subconscious mind which sits behind our mind and does the mischief. That is what subconscious mind is. It sits in the back and can spoil the image of human life by repeating experiences which have already been tasted and are recorded in the subconscious mind. So the subconscious mind must be taken care of and trained to be an aid to life.

Another pattern that must be confronted in Kundalini yoga is our self-belittlement and the feeling that we are very limited. "Oh, I, a poor humble self, can't do this. I am very miserable." We can play this game. There are three ways of playing it. Sometimes we play it to get sympathy from people, sometimes we play it to get recognized, and sometimes we really play it and we actually feel it. Everybody does it. It's just a matter of degree. Someone does it one percent, another does it one hundred percent. It means your activity in realizing your mental capacity is just that limited. You have not realized that your mind has an infinite horizon. There's actually no end to it.

Understand this today: There are no two people who are alike. Neither are they physically alike, nor are they mentally alike. They have only one likeness: The input of infinity can be equalized to the output of infinity. And that is the only thing in us which counts. We all can reach the state of infinity, of bliss, of nirvana. There are two hundred words for it. You can call it anything, it doesn't matter. But that's what it is.

Now I'll touch on a controversial point. Whatever religion you follow, no matter what you call it, you follow something meant for you to know your origin which is infinity. That religion should get rid of your self-belittlement and limitation and lift you to the full human capacity. Instead, what you usually end up knowing is prejudice, division of humanity, love and hatred on the basis of belonging to certain thoughts, or certain feelings, or certain practices. That has done more harm to humanity than the good the religions were intended to do. Today, we do not even understand the basic word "religion." It comes from *religio* and means looking back at your origin. And what is your origin? Spirit! And what is your end? Spirit! So what are you fighting about? What is the discussion? If you are constant and under all given circumstances you relate to one thing — that you are a part of infinity and you always lean on that power — then you'll never be unhappy. It is a practice.

We have never trained our minds to know our origin which is infinity. Instead we have run into rituals. All these churches, temples, and synagogues,

all the places of worship were meant to create group consciousness. We start with consciousness then progress to group consciousness and universal consciousness. These religious places were designed so that all the people believing one way could come and join together to praise the Lord and feel high. That was the purpose. But now people come there to fight elections and to think who should control the synagogue or church. Or the minister speaks and lays his number. It has become a regular mechanized ritual — a systematic system within the system. The purpose which was to get together to practice and feel and experience the group consciousness is gone. Man has become confused. For when a person does not have individual consciousness and does not develop that individual consciousness to a group consciousness, he cannot attain the universal consciousness. Barriers shall exist. And these are those barriers which keep a man limited. The development of group consciousness in the experience of infinity is the bridge to universal consciousness and the release of the unlimited self.

All the technology you need is in Kundalini yoga. But we have a mental sickness. We are not constant at anything. If you are very regular, if you practice so that you can cater to yourself and have a better experience, you will enjoy your life more and extend its length. Hopefully you will do your best. This knowledge and exchange is a brotherhood, it is a mutual existence. There's no big and no small. It's a sharing. It's very much a sharing. So if you are willing to get into that kind of sharing, that kind of love, that kind of existence, you are welcome. Otherwise, we are happy, you are happy. Wherever you are, you are; wherever we are, we are. There's no problem.

Man exists to help those who need existence. I always feel that pushing knowledge on people is pushing drugs. Pushing is pushing anyway, so I don't want to be a pusher of anything. That is something which I have never done in my life. I'm not going to push heavy knowledge on you, but I'd like to share with you certain things so that we can experience certain things.

In Kundalini Yoga the most important thing is experience. Your experience goes right into your heart. No words can be said because your consciousness will not accept them. Your mind may or may not. All we want to do is to extend your consciousness so you may have a wider horizon of grace and of knowing the truth. Then you can smoothly plan your life to any extent you like. You can radiate creativity and infinity in all aspects of your daily life.

Thank you very much for this evening. God bless you.

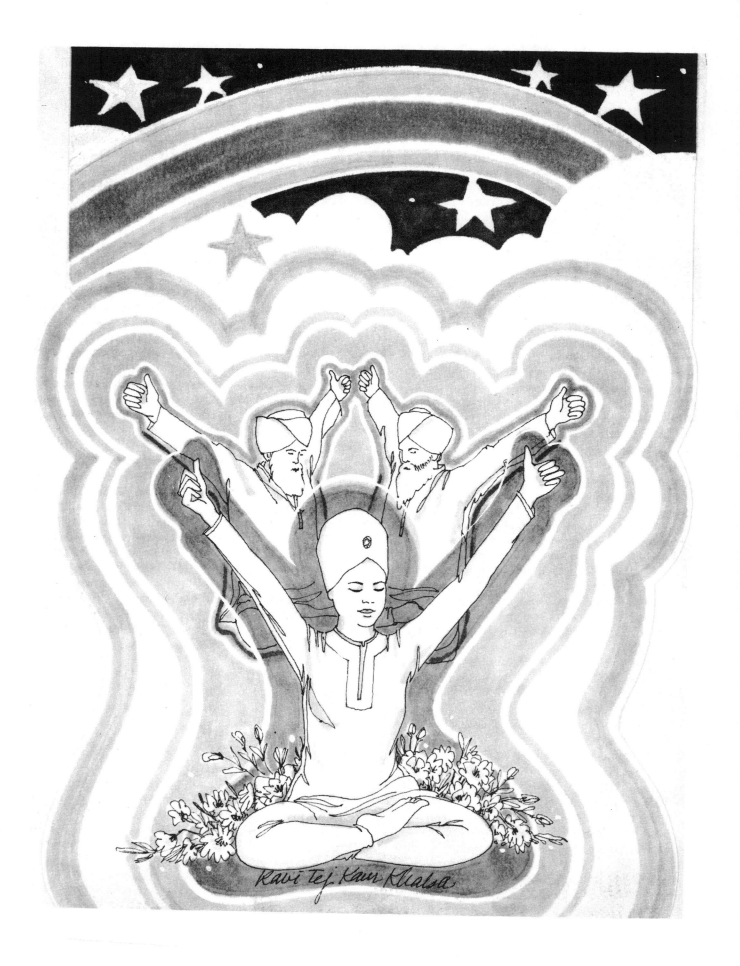

Ravi Tej Kaur Khalsa

Kundalini Yoga and Human Radiance

By Siri Singh Sahib Bhai Sahib

Harbhajan Singh Khalsa Yogiji

Tonight I would like you to ask any questions you like about Kundalini yoga, its nature or history.

Question: I have a friend who is a psychotherapist. He teaches Hatha yoga as part of his therapy. He was telling me that Kundalini yoga is an extremely dangerous form of yoga and can possibly lead to insanity if not handled right. Is this true?

Answer: It is very unfortunate that some people talk that way. First of all, they do not know what they are talking about. Second, they don't have any real experience of it. Actually, Kundalini yoga produces whole human beings, teachers, and yogis. A yogi is one who has a union with the supreme consciousness. Some people teach it as if it is a bunch of dumb exercises, but they have no right to call themselves yogis. If flexibility posture is the only yoga, then people in the circus are the best yogis.

Question: He doesn't consider himself a yogi. He just mentioned that he had thought that Kundalini yoga is a very dangerous aspect of yoga.

Answer: Ask him why he is practicing all the Hatha yoga postures. What is the purpose of Hatha yoga? The purpose of the Hatha yoga is to raise the awareness. It is a technology to bring the apana and prana, the moon and sun powers, together to raise the consciousness through the central equilibrium line. In other words, its stated aim is to raise the Kundalini. That is the purpose. But the problem is that it takes about 22 years to raise it that way even with perfect practice. That is the long method. It is a question of time only. Purpose is the same.

Teaching Hatha yoga and Kundalini yoga is very different. First of all, it is difficult to teach Kundalini yoga. A man who does not have a beam of energy within himself cannot teach it. That is the first fundamental. You have to be aware in consciousness. It is a matter of a level of consciousness. You should be at a certain steady level of consciousness to pull all the people up to that level. That is the real problem. You could come and I could give you a bunch of exercises. You would feel good, but when you talk about life and humanity and the total sum of existence and consciousness, then you have to feel that magnetism come out of me. If I can't give you that, there is nothing to pull you to that level. That is the basic difference.

Let's talk this way. Actually, there was a God. He uncoiled himself, opened himself up. This uncoiling process or manifestation process is known as Kundalini. What is dangerous about it? What is going to be uncoiled in you is *already* in you. It is an unlimited power and it is going to uncoil in you. There is danger when something outside is artificially put in you. But your system is already built to contain the energy of Kundalini. You simply are not utilizing that energy. If you start utilizing that energy, where is the danger? This talk of danger sometimes becomes the biggest danger and a big problem. All these yogis love me but they do not feel very good with me. They love me because, as a master of Kundalini yoga, it is very difficult to hate me. It takes a lot of strength to hate me. As a group we are a very powerful organization in the United States of America. We have a couple hundred thousand people. Name a large town, and there is a center nearby. The growth has all happened in three years.* It is basically very difficult to put down somebody with that kind of following and that kind of personality. Where is the root of the distrust and warnings? Why is Kundalini yoga put down? It is done either out of ignorance or simply because I teach it! It has never been taught publicity before. The other yogis feel guarded about the knowledge out of a sense of national and racial loyalty. You understand that India was conquered by the British people who were Christians. So the lower classes and working classes of India were converted to Christianity. Traditionally, in India, this class of people is called untouchable. The majority of the Christians came from the untouchables, so even now in their minds and hearts a Christian is still untouchable. They feel this great sovereign secret of Kundalini yoga was supposed to be learned only by highly special Brahmins. Now this Yogi Bhajan got hold of it and he is just freaking out and giving it to every American without discrimination. It is very dangerous. It is dangerous culturally.

When I went back to India where I lived for thirty-nine years, the one question everybody asked was, "What are you doing? What do you want to do in that country? Why are you teaching them?" All my friends were upset about it. They were not happy.

* 1969-1972, date of lecture

10

When I told them Americans have the potential to experience the infinity, they said, "Oh, no, no, no. What has gone wrong with you?" When they started questioning me, I withdrew and said, "Alright, I am happy with my Guru, what do I care. It is my destiny."

There are certain things in my life which I can't overcome. They are in my destiny. I never came to this country by my own choice. I had no means to reach all these people who have come to know me. People have come to me. I have never even thought or intellectualized for a moment and said, "I did it." What I feel is that those souls who have to come and learn from me are already in the body. I already have this knowledge which I am to share with them, so all I end up being is a postman to deliver their letters. When my mailbag is empty I can quit. That is how I feel.

What is Kundalini, actually? You experience it when the energy of the glandular system combines with the nervous system to create such a sensitivity that the totality of the brain receives signals and integrates them. Then a person understands the effect of the effect in a sequence of the causes. In other words, man becomes totally and wholly aware. We call it the yoga of awareness. Just as all rivers end up in the ocean, all yogas end up raising the kundalini in man. What is the kundalini? It is the creative potential of the man. In one year, about one hundred and thirty-five thousand people have practiced Kundalini yoga and we have heard no complaints whatsoever.

Somebody may want to talk out of jealousy or ignorance, but we don't have to answer to that. What is God consciousness? What is Christ consciousness? What you call Christ consciousness, we call Kundalini. When man uncoils his potential, in activity, that is what it is. When I started teaching Kundalini yoga everybody told me, "It will not be popular, you should start with Hatha yoga." I am a good Hatha yogi. When these Hatha yogis get sick, I treat them. I have a specialty in yoga therapy, where you use Hatha yoga postures and certain mudras and certain kriyas. But I chose not to teach just Hatha yoga. When I came to this country, I had to decide, "Am I going to do it for myself or am I going to do it for these people?" I felt that the people here needed the type of system which could give them a positive result in realization in a very short time. There is no better system known to me than Kundalini yoga. Raja yoga is very mental and a student has to be very prepared for it. The beauty of Kundalini yoga is that if you can just physically sit there with your pranayam automatically fixed, then with it, your mind is fixed. So a complete physical, mental and spiritual balance is achieved immediately in one kriya. That's why it works so effectively in a short time. To achieve universal consciousness through any method you have to raise your kundalini.

To do this, a little technology and science is needed. After the eighth year of life, the pineal gland does not secrete fully. It needs to get the reserve energy that is stored at your belly-button area, the navel point. That energy which developed you and gave you this shape and brought you on this earth has absolutely no residue. It is a pure energy. Do you understand what I am saying? That pure energy is still there. All you have to do is uncoil that energy and make a functional connection with your pineal gland. Once that master gland, the seat of the soul, has started secreting, it will give you the power to reach your self-realization in relationship to the total universal awareness. Scientifically speaking, that is what must happen. But some people are still ignorant. If I would have talked a hundred years ago about atomic energy people would have said, "Oh, it is dangerous. It is impossible. Who wants to do that?" First of all they didn't know about the atom. It is a human problem, not an individual problem. Without knowing anything about what something is or what something actually means, we have opinions. Not only do we have opinions, but we have *set* opinions!

Occasionally you will find an awareness which is unique in certain people who may not be practicing Kundalini yoga but are known as having a sixth sense. They have inborn capacities. They have some intuitive power which tells them that the consequences of certain sequences of actions will be disastrous in the end. If you have this intuitive relationship between the individual consciousness and universal consciousness, you can compute what someone is trying to say before they say it. What they actually say is unimportant. You will know what they intend and what they mean. It is not very difficult. If a man comes to you, you may not even let him talk. You just say, "Well, you have come and you are ultimately going to ask me for a hundred dollars, but friend, I don't have it." I used to do that sometimes but people started sending word that I am a great psychic. That is not a good reputation so now I am very quiet about it. This intuitive capacity is natural. Actually, you become sensitive to the auric radiance of another person. As the signal comes, all you have to do is compute it and you will know what he is talking about. His words do not mean anything. You already know what he means. Most people are not aware that they have this ability in them. But with a little mental work, it can be achieved.

Our life as it is today has one basic human problem. We have to understand: A is A, B is B, C is C. Because C doesn't understand what C is, he cannot understand what B is and what A is. And that is the total conflict in this world and it is a source of unhappiness to the human being. If C understands what C is, in that understanding his relationship with B and with A will be very clear, and there will be no place for doubt. Since C doesn't understand what C is, C doesn't understand what B is either, but he does want to express himself about

B and A. This kind of expression which is not based on a clear understanding will always misguide. That is why this world has become a puzzle to us. Actually, the world is very clear. We are all human beings on this planet. We are supposed to live with each other in love, work as a worship and follow the path of righteousness, goading our lives through the time cycle of human energy to get across to infinity.

Why do we not fit in, in spite of the fact that we have the ability to fit in? There may be an ordinary man who is a grade B medical student. He gets a great opportunity. He rises above everything to the top. Then there may be a doctor who is a very brilliant student at college, but he never gets the opportunity. The confusion occurs when in spite of our equipped personality, we sometimes do not thrive and we do not understand why. There is a way to make sense out of this. We understand it intuitively, but scientifically it takes a little time.

According to the yogis, the symbol of man is the arc of life that we call an aura. The human aura is the arc of life. It is brilliant and white. Human existence depends on that arc. Most people can't see it and can't understand it. If you can see it, you can recognize the state of disease as well as the abilities of a person. All energy in existence has its own cycle just as this human being has his own cycle. That's what makes a human being unique. Every magnetic field has to cross this magnetic field of your arc line. The strength of the magnetic field of your arc determines how the other magnetic fields can or cannot enter and affect you.

Now a question arises. If there is a positive opportunity or vibration, will this arc of light reflect it so it won't enter? No! That positive energy will merge in it and will relate to the earth. If it is negative, it will be cancelled out at the arc line. Any person whose mental vibraton results in a strong arc will protect all fragile areas of his life automatically with that arc.

When the magnetic field is strong, you relate to emotions differently. You can choose to relate to someone or disconnect from their influence. When your radiance is strong and you direct it to someone, they will want to talk to you and be around you in spite of great differences or pains. When man has the energy and he has the power through his psyche to relate or to forget, then he has nothing to worry about. The projection of his magnetic field will arrange the rays of his existence so that his psycho-electro-magnetic circle can organize all the surrounding magnetic fields in tune. In other words, the environment will operate in tune with his purpose.

Let me say this in spiritual language. When the divine source that prevails through the man projects out the light of God, all darkness will go away. Wherever he shall go, there shall be light, beauty, bounty and fulfillment. These two explanations are the same, but one is in mystic language and the other is in scientific language. Kundalini yoga is the science of changing and strengthening the radiance to give expanded life and capacity.

I'll give you an example of understanding human behavior with these two languages. Whenever the individual consciousness, while radiating, feels a cut or dip in the area of radiance, the connection that is trying to be made is not complete. When there is a cut, you cannot radiate correctly and the cycle of energy cannot complete itself into a creative action. What is a cut? A cut is division of energy.

Question: Well, what would cause a cut like this?

Answer: I am coming to that. We all have set patterns of behavior on which the pattern of consciousness is based. These patterns hold our personalities. A Hindu, for example, cannot eat meat because in his consciousness he feels it is a sin. A Muslim cannot eat pork because in his consciousness he feels it is a sin. A Christian eats meat and pork, because in his consciousness it is not a sin. Your consciousness must form a pattern of flow. Once you fix the pattern and frequency of that flow, then any time that your needs conflict with that established pattern, you cannot radiate. That's why some people cannot look into your eyes and talk, and others don't like to face you. What is wrong? Nothing, but a pattern of flow has been set. It is a combination of social environment and inner environment that forms the patterns. Those patterns form cavities in the aura. A cavity in consciousness is a duality. We act but we know that we don't think about it. Whenever your intellect, the giver of the thoughts, does not correspond to your set behavior, you have a problem.

In a church, we would say that this is the conflict of a sinful man. What happens when you go and confess to a minister? What does he give you? Does he have some key to bind you up? You pour yourself out and he tells you that you are forgiven. You have a set pattern of belief in him; therefore, you can believe him and you can go on. Whenever something bothers you, there is only one way to get out of it. You have to have a captain, *you have to have a person who will not betray your faith and who will counsel you to return to the path of righteousness.* In other words, he should set the flow of the psyche in tune with the surrounding magnetic field. In mystic or spiritual language, we say that a man who has committed a sin comes and confesses in the house of the Lord and the Lord accepts his prayers and blesses him to the light. He again starts living in a bountiful world. The two explanations are exactly the same. In this modern world, when there is a problem, people go to the psychiatrist who drinks coffee and has the patience to listen to them and to make them talk. Then through his experience he tells them that they have to work out the whole thing, cautiously. By charging a couple of thousand dollars, the psychiatrist makes the guy alert to the idea that he has to stop somewhere and solve his own problem. He has to put in an effort. This is what motivates him. It is not the psychiatrist, it is not the priest in the church. It is your acceptance of the environmental behaviors and the urge to look back to your basic origin and start understanding that you are the creative source and nucleus of the whole vibratory effect in which you live. The moment you understand this, you are alright, there's no problem. The moment you know you are you, the problem is solved. When you understand who and what you are, your radiance projects in the universal radiance and everything becomes creative around you. This confirmed relationship of responsiveness in consciousness between the finite self and the infinite self is the gift of Kundalini.

What is the problem that arises between a father and son? Is there any father who wants to denounce his son? No. If he does denounce him, what forces him to? Some action of the son. If a father wants to accept his son, what makes his son the most acceptable? Action. But action at what level? The action must be at the father's level of consciousness. If the father is a hunter and a fisherman, and the son goes and fishes and brings home a lot of fishes, the father says, "Oh my, I'm impressed!" Suppose instead the son used to go for eight hours and get two fishes. If he starts telling his father, "Fishing is no good. It is just killing the life in the ocean for no reason. Don't do it. You can't even create one fish but destroy as many as you can hook. How can you kill all those poor beautiful things in the ocean?" The father will get angry and say, "Okay. You get off my back and hit the road. Eat your own bread. Get out of my house and keep going. I don't want to listen to you." He will react this way because he can't understand the son's point of view.

What is our understanding? It's our pattern of behavior. What is a pattern of behavior? It is the rate of frequency and the radiance of the psyche and the magnetic field in relationship to the universal psyche and magnetic force. If you can relate with that universal radiation so the beam and frequency of projection is clear, then you have communicated with the universe and it will support you just as a happy father will support his son, his creation. *This relationship of consciousness to the infinite consciousness is the one fundamental requirement of life and the aim of yoga.*

There once was a businessman who wanted to find a man to manage his stores. He advertised. Everybody came with great experience and recommendations. The last interview was with a man who had no experience. The businessman said, "Why don't you have any recommendations?" He said, "Sir, if you want to recruit someone with a recommendation, you have already interviewed many. Just select one. But if you ever need a man, remember me and do call me. Thank you very much." He left smiling. The businessman started thinking. Is a manager a man or is a man a manager? He sat on this problem for one week and finally came to a con-

clusion. A perfect manager may not be a man in the sense of activity. He discussed it with one of his friends. His friend said, "What are you talking about? That man just said I am a man, and you started believing him. What about his recommendations? These other people have already worked as managers of stores." The owner said, "They are managers of stores, but none of them could tell me that he is a man. I'd like to try this man." So he called him. He said, "Alright. You manage my store." The man said, "Sir, I have a problem. It is true I am a man. If you make a manager out of me then I'll manage the stores. My problem is that I am only a man, I am not yet a manager." The businessman asked, "How can I train you in all those skills?" The man replied, "It is nothing. If you will just work for fifteen days as a manager, I will watch you and I will know." So the owner worked for fifteen days and this guy picked up everything. He was perfect. Sometime later they were sitting together and the owner asked, "I would like to understand something. How can you have all my confidence so that I trust you to do everything perfectly? You are not a very qualified man. Your only training was seeing me work for fifteen days." The new manager said, "Sir, one thing you must understand. I only know one thing: 'I am, I am.' My consciousness is very clear about the words 'I am, I am!' When anything bothers me, I tell myself one thing: 'I am, I am,' and I get to it. The moment you know you are you, there is no problem."

The basic unit of you is equal to your radiance plus your activity. That radiance is the mind and the activity is the gross. Let me express this in the mystic sense. When the soul opens up the heart, man becomes divine. You may say it any way you like. A man has to understand his existence in relationship to the universe. Whosoever understands this knows the truth. The whole world around you will be beautiful if you understand that you are you. In all walks of your life remember you are you. *"I am, I am."* That is the mantra. The Kundalini and Kundalini yoga are very natural elements that rapidly make you what you already are and bring you to the practical experience of infinity.

Morning Sadhana

The Foundation of a Spiritual Life

By M.S.S. Gurucharan Singh Khalsa

This is the dawning of the Age of Aquarius. It is the cusp period of the time. It is the end of the adolescence of mankind. But every adolescent experiences growing pains and periods of struggle to adjust to his adult potentials. In the next few decades, we will experience tremendous sociological, psychological, and physical changes. Our sense of who we are, what our responsibilities are, and what our potentials are will shift radically. Instead of man viewing himself as a finite piece of dust, glorified with grand delusions, man shall see himself as an intricate and finite physical vessel linked to an infinite source of universal consciousness and energy. The tide of our evolution will wash away the old concepts of individuality and establish new priorities in life. The meaning and stability of life will focus on the harmony between the individual psyche and the universal psyche. We will strive to create lifestyles which unleash our highest potentials and serve a global and cosmic consciousness. The foundation of these new lifestyles will be *sadhana*: a disciplined practice to integrate body, mind, and spirit.

The techniques taught by Siri Singh Sahib Bhai Sahib Harbhajan Singh Khalsa Yogiji are an important part of forming the new age culture. The techniques of Kundalini yoga and the lifestyle and discipline of the Sikh Dharma offer an effective and efficient way to build the potential of each person in the context of humility and service to the whole body of mankind. The first teaching of this lifestyle is to rise before dawn every day and do a sadhana. The importance of doing sadhana has been emphasized by every major discipline of consciousness that has been used successfully by people to better themselves and the societies in which they live. It cannot be overemphasized. It should not be overlooked. The symbol for the Age of Aquarius is the bearer of truth. Its motto is "I know, therefore I believe." So it demands a practical personal experience to verify the ancient spiritual truths. To build the experience within yourself requires constant practice and a commitment to your higher consciousness.

The following discussion and guidelines of sadhana are offered as clarification of the techniques and not as an absolute dictum intended to limit its form. There must always be inspiration at the heart of any real sadhana, and that precludes a rigid structure.

PROCESS AND PROGRESS IN SADHANA

The essence of the progress and direction of sadhana is in the sequence *sadhana, aradhana,* and *prabhupati,* or roughly translated: discipline, attitude, and aptitude or mastery. Sadhana is the overall practice as well as a part of the process. The steps are really inseparable.

To understand the first step which is daily sadhana, you must see it within the context of aradhana and prabhupati. *Sadhana* means any practice of self correction that provides the mind and body with a disciplined channel to express the infinite within one's self. It is a practice that resets your cycles and patterns to the rhythm of your ultimate aims. It is a time each day to notice all the negative habits that lead you away from higher consciousness and to eliminate the desires

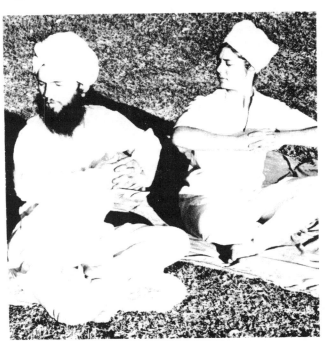

underlying those habits one by one. This is a conscious activity. You consciously choose to wake up in the early hours of the morning instead of sleeping. You consciously exercise the body and exalt the infinite in your heart with your voice and attitude. Each day is different. Each day, you are different. Every 72 hours all the cells of your body totally change. Sickness comes and goes. Motivation waxes and wanes. But through all the flux of life, through all the variations of our minds and palpitations of unsure hearts, we consciously choose to maintain a constant and regular practice. By this commitment we establish a priority in life above all the changes: to exalt the infinite universal self in order to develop our finite selves as better channels to express unlimited nature.

The yogic scriptures require at least 2-1/2 hours of sadhana before the rising of the sun. You must dedicate at least one-tenth of each day to God. It is in these hours that the auric protection and guidance of the teacher is most prevalent to all who wish to meditate. It is in these hours that the *prana*, the basic life force of consciousness, concentrates and the physical cleansing is accomplished more easily in these hours than during the rest of the day. Few people are awake and busy, so the clutter and bustle of daily activities does not interfere with you.

Though many challenges may come to stop your constant early morning practice, as you conquer each one, you will build your will power, your confidence, and the ability to beam your mind. This constancy linked with the natural circadian rhythm of the sun provides rhythm in your life. This is no small accomplishment. If at the same time each day, you tune all your mental and physical rhythms to each other, then no part of yourself will be out of step with any other part of yourself. The entire day flows better. Besides this, a natural rhythm associated with any activity helps you to learn that activity better. If you try to learn a particular task at the same time each day, you will learn it more efficiently. If you learn to meditate at the same time every day, it becomes easier and easier.

In meditation, you are cleaning the subconscious of fears and releasing new reservoirs of consciousness and energy to guide you. As each fear comes up and you look upon it neutrally, the fear loses its power over you. You become more flexible and feel more free. Most fears were learned at a particular time of day. So, these fears tend to occur most intensely at the time of day they were experienced. By meditating at sadhana time, you slowly attract the anxieties from all other parts of the day. Normally you react to anxieties on their time and on their conditions. In meditation the effects of old fears come to you on your time and under your conditions. Since they come at the same time each day, it becomes easier and easier to deal with each one. Eventually the mind is cleared of the clouds of fear and begins to see the light and power of creative consciousness. Then the morning meditation clears out the daily worries and projections so no further long-term subconscious fears can accumulate.

After practicing a regular sadhana for some time, the teachings and consciousness begin to seep into the deeper parts of the mind. This period of time may be 40 days or one and one-half years. It depends on the individual, the intensity of effort, and the starting condition. The efforts which you consciously planted have grown roots, and the offshoots are able to stand on their own. The subconscious mind finally gets your message. It understands that you are sincere, that meditation is a priority, that every day at this time you begin to wake up automatically without the aid of an alarm, and that even when traveling you will meditate every day on time. The subconscious begins to support you and sadhana begins to feel effortless. The subconscious, which directs about 60% of our activities and responses by habit, has now acquired a habit to have the consciousness of sadhana.

In the beginning, the conscious efforts of sadhana may seem like a negative activity. It imposes discipline at the cost of some other activities such as sleep. It makes you deal with the many influences that resist your attempts to be regular. But as sadhana becomes aradhana, there can only be positive feeling left as a result of experience. You have established a channel that allows the awakened desires of your higher mind to connect with the universal self. During this period, the mind becomes more active in its subconscious cleaning. If you find resistance now it is not from the fast flux of external changes. You confront a basic question: Are you willing to act and think in your highest consciousness, or do you want to hang on to your old identity even longer? If the choice is for the higher self, then sadhana becomes a joy and you leap up each morning to meet it. If you put off the decision, you will feel motivated, then unmotivated; you will feel more tired or sick than you may be to avoid getting up; and you may even fall asleep whenever you meditate, in an attempt to avoid this commitment to your self. A major pitfall at this stage is the feeling that you have "made it." Since the physical habit is firmly established, you become lax in the mental discipline of beaming the mind to the infinite. It is just like climbing a mountain: when you reach a high plateau, your impulse is to camp and look at the valleys below. You want to dine on succulent berries and rest from the strenuous climb. But waiting too long makes the muscles slack and soon you may even forget why you wanted to climb to the top when this level is so comfortable. You know the rest of the climb is harder, narrower, and colder than what you have already experienced. So you resist the last step. This is an apt metaphor for climbing the heights of selfhood. When we have practiced enough to confirm an attitude, we relax. We make it to sadhana, but fall asleep. We will

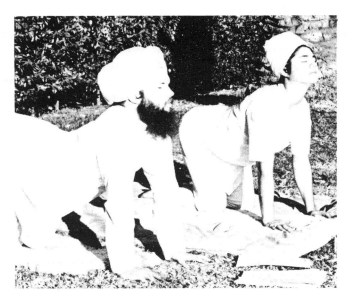

chant the Nam, but sometimes feel the words are just mechanical motions without meaning because we lose touch with our initial motivations. This is part of the subconscious reorganization that affects motivation and intent. At some point in this, you may feel absolutely no motivation to do what you have set out to do and are doing. It is then that the regular habit of sadhana and the earlier commitments are essential. The thought of duty and of the Nam itself may become your only reasons for continuing. If you are constant through this dark time, you can tap new sources of energy and strength within yourself. You will build a dependence directly on the infinite and never need to rely on a finite motivation or structure for the sense of self, for the sense of meaningfulness, or for the power to act creatively.

Once aradhana has cleaned the subconscious and confirmed your motivation to know, merge, and use the infinite, you enter into *prabhupati*, or mastery of God. This is the state of neutrality. Your motivation is neutral. No finite thing motivates you. No money, no fame, no sex, no personal advancement is enough to determine your actions. You cease to be manipulated by things. Most of us are so attached to our possesions and hopes that we cannot creatively and freely act in the highest consciousness of each moment. We compromise our potential to possess our past. In this neutral state, you sense the infinite in all things. Nothing motivates you except the sense of the infinite existence itself. Motivation comes from the center of your being.

The stage of prabhupati represents the opening and atunement to the superconsciousness. The conscious mind has merged with the subconscious mind, and there is no conflict in the personality. Everything is experienced as a harmony even if the gross outward circumstance seems challenging or disastrous. A person feels more of the pain of the entire cosmos, and more of its joy, but rests in the neutral and sublime state of mind — *mastery of God.*

It is the full awakening and integration of compassion into the personality. Compassion gives man a capacity to forgive the unforgivable. God is bound to maintain the Law of Polarity throughout the cosmos. If ill acts are created, then ill acts must be received. If you steal, He must steal from you. This gives order and law to the world. Since these laws govern the events of normal life, the time we live in acts to teach us to come in accordance with universal law and God's will. A man in prabhupati is an exception. He can go beyond the laws of time and polarity into the state of compassion. He can forgive a thief who has robbed him, and even plant in that person the inspiration to reach the infinite. An example of this is the story of Balmikhi.

Balmikhi was a thief and a head-cutter with an excellent reputation for efficiency and success. No one ever passed Balmikhi's hiding spot without getting his head parted from his body and his coin placed in the head-cutter's pocket. For generations his whole family had been taught this skill. With diligent study, he became the best of all. People who knew of his reputation stayed away. Even the king's men did not challenge him.

On this particular day a traveling holy man who had not heard the stories walked by the robber's lair. Balmikhi jumped him with raised sword. To his surprise, the saint kneeled with bowed head and thanked the thief slyly, "You are most generous to give me my day of liberation, kind thief. I have waited long to leave this physical body. Please hurry so I may join the Creator!" The thief never had a client who uttered such a strange plea. He raised his sword to accomodate the plea when the holy man exclaimed, "Wait! As a truthful being I must be fair to you and not leave this world in a half-truth. If you kill me then you will die within three days. Now you know. Please go ahead."

This perturbed Balmikhi. He knew that saints' words always come true since the power of God lives in their tongues. He held back the fatal cut and asked, "I know what you say will come to pass. Is there no way to escape this destiny?" The saint replied, "If one of your family will voluntarily die at the same time I do, you will be spared. But I do not think they love you that much."

Balmikhi tied up the saint and went to his house. He called together his entire clan and explained the situation. "I must kill this holy man to uphold my reputation. I have supported you all for years with my special skills. Now who of you loves me enough to sacrifice for me?" No one moved forward to confirm his confidence in their love. He pleaded again and again. When he realized he could persuade no one, he returned to the holy man. He sat next to the saint and loosened his bonds. He became very depressed. His mind fogged over with memories of all he had done. He felt a basic lack of understanding about life. He was never taught how to love, how to be loved, and how to be spiritually great.

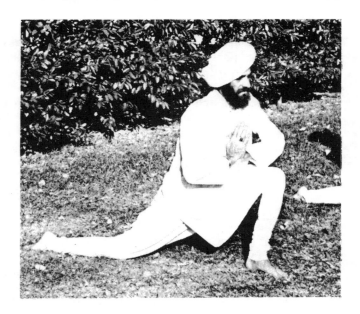

The saint saw his perplexed condition. He saw the ignorance surrounding the man and his sincere desire to understand the truth. The great saint got into a state of compassion. With a touch of his fingers to the thief's forehead he cleared the subconscious of its fears and ignorance. The thief looked up with clear eyes in blissful devotion. He said, "Great man, you have given me the vision of my inner infinity. Now give me a practice of sadhana so I can confirm this consciousness and teach its freedom to others." The holy man gave Balmikhi a kriya. Balmikhi sat for three days without moving and went deep into the meditation. The same discipline and alertness he used to become a master thief and head-cutter was now applied with force and sincerity to his new goal. The same energy that made him a thief now made him a saint. In later years, he taught thousands the liberated life and has been remembered even to this day.

Compassion is the highest virtue. It can remake even the lowest part of the creation into the highest of God's creatures. In acts of compassion a kind of vacuum is created, for the law of action and reaction has been transcended. Nature does not love a vacuum and neither does God. So he rushes to the service of that saint who has the compassion to serve. God must assist that consciousness which is the expression of the highest exalted form of God Himself.

During the years when Guru Nanak lived a householder's life, he was in charge of a storehouse which issued grain to the Nawab's servants in Sultanpur. For three years he gave grain to all who asked for it, according to their need.

A rumor came to the Nawab that Nanak was recklessly giving away grain and that the royal stores were now empty. The Nawab ordered an investigation. Very carefully the records were checked and the grain was weighed. Not only was the storehouse full of grain, but there was even more than was to be expected. It is said that as Nanak counted out the measures of grain he would reach the number thirteen and endlessly repeat its name, *"taira,"* which also means "yours." He would say, "Yours, O God, I am yours." as he gave away all the grain. In a trance-like ecstasy, he always distributed more than was stored.

Guru Nanak's service to the people in compassionately filling their needs created a "vacuum," an empty storehouse which was then filled by the One who gives everything.

In prabhupati every moment of the day is a realized sadhana. There is no moment you are asleep and unaware of the present and requirements of the universal consciousness. You cease to do what is right for you and do only that which is right for all.

The experience of sadhana is a daily initiation. No one in 3HO ever initiates anyone into a kriya or secret mantra. We feel there is no secret between man and God, so there should be no secret between man and man about God. The way to the infinite is clear. It is open to all. It is clouded only by our own ignorance, fears and lack of discipline. To take an initiation means to make a confirmed beginning. Every morning in sadhana, you bow before the infinite. Your higher self initiates your lower self and that is the secret of all secrets. The whole world assists you in this daily initiation. As you begin sadhana there is nothing around you except darkness. Worldly activity is at a minimum. As you sit and meditate on the infinite Creator, the day slowly dawns. Every cell of your being learns that exalting the Name leads from darkness to light. The entire subconscious is alert to the primal experience of dawn and senses a rebirth. The mind projects sensitivity and trust of the higher self's demands and is led past its ignorance and error to enlightened vision. To realize this is true initiation.

The man who practices a perfect sadhana begins to glow. He gains the ability to guide and inspire others. Just being in his presence helps clear your mind of useless conflicts. He has opened the guiding potential of his supermind in his aura.

MENTAL STRUCTURE

Each person has an individual mind. Its experience and understanding is limited by the structures that have formed it: culture, upbringing, samskaras, physical capacity of the body, etc. In order to grow and be able to integrate its experience, the individual mind must experience the universal mind. Every experience the individual mind has of the universal mind contributes to the growth of a guiding consciousness or supermind. Every sadhana that contacts the infinite builds the supermind. Your auric radiance increases and others who come within your presence begin to experience that supermind and guidance as well.

There are two main ways to connect the individual mind to the universal mind and build the supermind. The first method is *pratyahar*. In this method you inject the universal mind into the individual mind by a contraction process. You watch each thought pattern that enters the mind. You choose between them on the basis of whether it takes you to the infinite or not. You substitute a positive thought for each negative one so you become neutral or at least positive. If you have desires in the individual mind that require action, use the will to act only on those that are universal. Once this choice becomes automatic you are practicing pratyahar. Everything will lead you to connect and draw energy from the universal mind to the individual mind.

The second method is *Laya*. The word itself means devotion, absorption and levitation. The process suspends the self directly in a sense of the infinite rather than by finding the infinite starting with finite things. In Laya yoga techniques, you recognize nothing in yourself except the infinite. These techniques always involve the use of mantra with a special breathing rhythm. The breathing allows the mind to release particular emotional and intuitive energies that power the consciousness to expand. In this technique you go from the individual mind to the universal mind.

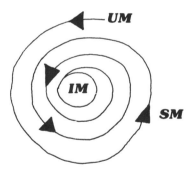

PRATYAHAR

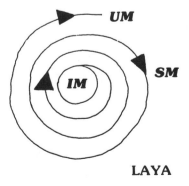

LAYA

IM — *Individual Mind*
SM — *Super Mind*
UM — *Universal Mind*

Most of the problems of contemporary society do not stem from sex, guilt, power, etc. The basic problem is a loss of the sense of meaning and value in the individual self. The cultural beliefs and religious symbols that were once very vital to us and acted as a supermind have been divested of their potency. To reestablish our values so that we can focus on goals that fulfill our potentials, we must reconnect with our own inner creative nature. The practice of sadhana to stimulate the superconscious is the key to this.

The practical effect of the supermind is to change the perception of all ordinary things in the individual's life. It invests everything with the self. It prepares the ground for self-realization. The supermind sees a tree as a tree, but also as a symbol of life and patient growth. All parts of life become a lesson and a guide to the individual mind. The world becomes the mirror of self, as your self becomes the image of God. Problems in all parts of life become smaller and the inherent integrative and creative powers of our psyche are freed to operate and produce harmony.

GROUP SADHANA AND THE EXPANDED SELF

Sadhana is a discipline that moves us toward cosmic consciousness and self realization. To reach that high state of prabhupati, we must master the intermediate state of group consciousness. A practice and testing ground for this is the ashram community.

A 3HO Kundalini Yoga Ashram and Sikh Dharma Training Center has two basic forces in operation: the techniques of Kundalini yoga and the lifestyle of the Sikh Dharma. The yoga techniques stimulate the basic evolutionary force in the psyche. From this the urge to grow increases. Each person feels the expansion of his own energy or *shakti*. As his energy increases he can see its effects in the ability to influence people, channelize the will, and be sensitive to subtle energies. It is possible that the experience of expansion can lead to a great spiritual ego which is less curable than cancer! The Sikh humility and respect for the one Creator blocks that. The House of Guru Ram Das puts the ideals of self-sacrifice, service, and humility into daily practice.

It is important for a practitioner of a powerful discipline not to become too self-involved. If all the energy developed and released in sadhana were focused through our own ego structure, we could become imbalanced and narcissistic. The scale of ego development of a yogi has five steps. The lowest is that of egomania. Here everything is valueless unless it corresponds to the individual desire. There is no sympathy or understanding for another person. The second step is that of egotism. A person in this stage is not as relentless in his ego. He appears arrogant rather than maniacal. He is aware of other egos as well as his own but chooses himself. The third step is that of ego-centeredness. Here the person is consciously developing his capacities. He may include others in his existence but his main experiences are in the realm of emotion and action. His perspective will be limited. The fourth step is self-centeredness. This stage is often mistaken for the last step. The person transcends the rigid barrier of ego and identifies in experience with a larger sense of self. He begins to realize that his capacity is beyond that normally available to the ego. This is often a pleasant vision of the self, full of discovery and excitement. The last step is the stage of selflessness. Every identity of the self is still limited as before. There exists a broader but finite ego. But in this final step there is a merger with the practical sense of infinity. This is experienced in terms of service. The selfless person becomes an observer, even of his own actions. He has neutrality and equanimity. If he wants to rid himself of depression, he helps cure others of the malady. The stage of selflessness gives the ability to forgive the past and live in harmony with the cosmos. This final stage of growth is seldom reached individually. It requires the test and support of a group.

By living in a group that shares the same teachings, lifestyle, and consciousness, it is very difficult to do some spurious action that denies your new consciousness. Everyone, or at least someone, will notice and give you the proper feedback and encouragement to help you keep to your dharma. Remember, as much as we like to change instantly, the subconscious mind and old patterns form at least 60% of our actions. A strong group helps you to train that deep part of the mind. In an ashram community, you become used to making decisions that benefit the entire group instead of just yourself. This lays the foundation for becoming an enlightened leader.

Doing sadhana in a group develops a higher interpersonal sensitivity in the community. At the beginning of sadhana everyone has a different vibration. Some have traces of dreams, others are already filled with concerns for the day, and still others come with different expectations about sadhana. The more people there are the more these individual differences balance and cancel each other out. The happiness of one person balances the sadness of another. Then the entire group finds its energy directed by the activity of the sadhana itself. The individual auras merge and form a group aura. If the group is well tuned into the infinite, a rainbow aura forms that reflects all colors. A bluish color of sincerity and devotion predominates. One hour of sharing this type of energy can erase the effects of a week of arguments and discord. The strength of a community is directly proportional to the strength of their group sadhana. This auric

transformation aids the practitioner in making the step beyond ego centeredness.

By the end of morning sadhana, when everyone's energy has intermingled and merged, it is easy to communicate and be on the "same wavelength." You see this effect throughout the day. There will be fewer misunderstandings in the area of communications.

An ashram is the center of the community. It is where everyone gathers in the early morning hours. Literally, it means "house of the teacher." Its residents are servants and teachers of that higher consciousness. If the ashram is to serve its function in actively relating and adding to the community, a strong group sadhana is essential. If everyone did an individual sadhana, the power of unity would be lost and the individuals would only move toward ego- or self-centered activity.

If you are not in an ashram community, see if there is a local ashram where you can practice or get a few friends or members of your family to practice with you.

THE PRACTICAL STRUCTURE OF SADHANA

Knowing the mental and spiritual process of sadhana is not enough. The essence of a good sadhana is constant practice. Nothing, absolutely nothing, replaces the value and effects of practice. Without it, all studies, writings, and hopes become empty and meaningless.

There are many kinds of sadhanas, but there is a practical structure in a sadhana to give the optimal results. There are special sadhanas for people who have special psychological and physical problems. We will only describe some ideal structures for a complete sadhana that apply to physically and mentally normal yogic enthusiasts. The models can appy to an individual sadhana, but they are written for a group sadhana.

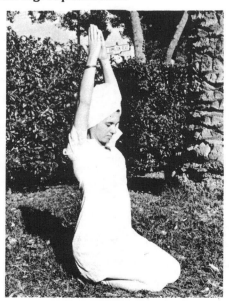

There are five main steps to building a complete sadhana.

PHYSICAL ENVIRONMENTS

It is difficult to imagine someone who would choose to do a sadhana next to a busy street. It is possible, but choosing that environment is certainly not an aid to normal meditation. In a meditative sadhana you become supersensitive and the environment that surrounds you has a huge effect on the ease of going into meditation. Colors, sounds and even the past usage of the room all register in your consciousness and affect its energy. There are rooms beautifully designed and used only for meditation; just walking in one is inspired to meditate, as being in the forest of the High Sierras automatically draws us into a meditative state.

The first step is to choose a place that is used mainly or entirely for sadhana. It should always be kept perfectly clean and neat. Arrange pictures and other objects that represent higher consciousness aesthetically around the room. If you are blessed with *Siri Guru Granth Sahib** in your ashram or home, a separate room should be provided. If this is not possible, then a curtain enclosing the *Guru Granth Sahib,* or some other appropriate form of separation from the rest of the room is necessary. The meditation room should smell fresh. Air should be allowed to circulate and the temperature should be moderate. Too much cold may harm the body in deep meditations. Too much heat will induce sleep and poor circulation. The spot you sit on should be covered with an animal skin or a wool blanket since they are non-static and insulate your psycho-electromagnetic field from the electromagnetic field of the earth. If a skin or proper fabric is unavailable, the next best substance to sit on is wood. As you become calm through meditation, you become more sensitive to the waves of energy within and without. Before meditation you may have required a high level of constant change and stimulation to be alert. Now stimulation from the inner self is enough. Sharp noises and constant interruptions should be minimized during meditation and sadhana. In some stages of meditation a closing door may sound like an explosion. For a graceful meditation choose a graceful environment.

PHYSICAL SELF

Create some kind of purification ritual that you never fail to perform. Wake yourself gently in the morning and do the standard wake-up exercises.* Remember to drink a few glasses of water. Take either a cold shower or a cold-warm-cold shower while chanting songs of divine praise. Let the clear

*Wake-up exercises at end of article.

flow of the water clean your aura of nighttime thoughts. Stimulate your circulation to flush the residues of nocturnal cleansing out of your body. You cannot meditate fully if your circulation is still in patterns suited for sleep or drowsiness. Massage the whole body, especially the feet, hands, face and ears while in the shower. If you are extra kind to yourself use some almond oil on the skin. A turban or house turban should be worn by men after the bath, and at least a chuni or scarf by women. Put on clothing which is loose and flexible but which is neat and clean. White is the best color for sadhana clothes. Do not wear the same garments to sadhana as you wore to bed. You must tell your consciousness in every way that you can that sadhana is a special activity that you prepare for and even dress specially, for your mind will be more alert and far more cooperative if it knows an important event is about to take place. Choose a meditation blanket or shawl made of wool, silk, or cotton. Use it only for meditation. Over a period of time the shawl will absorb the vibrations of sadhana. Then just putting it on will immediately aid your efforts.

MENTAL ENVIRONMENTS.

If all the physical preparations have been cared for, make sure that you set your mind for group consciousness. If you are leading the sadhana, check for unexpected visitors and guests. If they do not know your procedure, make them secure with a brief explanation. Make sure anything that is said is very positive. If your thoughts are positive and creative in the morning you will feel good all day.

Clearly establish who is to start the sadhana. The more people in the group the better. When you chant by yourself you are only one voice, but sitting with others the effect of your sound is multiplied by adding to the sound of others and by others hearing and reflecting your voice. If you must do sadhana by yourself, then while you are chanting imagine a million others all around you. Hear them all chanting with yourself in the middle not moving at all. Feel that you do not chant physically and yet are leading the chant and letting the chant lead you. As you imagine this, continue chanting.

MENTAL SELF

The most important step is to realize the presence of the teacher. Chant *"Ong Namo Guru Dev Namo,"* and feel the inflow of energy and light to your body and mind. Meditate on your higher teacher and feel that in all devotion and humility you are asking for guidance in sadhana. Pray that no matter how feeble your effort may be, the maximum benefit will be returned to help you serve humanity in the will of the Creator. Realize at this point that no student is the teacher. During sadhana the only teacher is the Guru. Awaken yourself consciously to the fact that you do not know what the results of your efforts will be and dedicate the results to the infinite.

Many people build a regular sadhana but fall into the pit of boredom. They become bored because of false expectations. They want an experience of flashing light and sparking energy. Although this does occur at times, it is more important to expect contact with the infinite. Let the infinite determine what form the connection will take. Realize that doing the same chant or the same exercise you have done many times before can give you a totally different effect *today*. Today is the beginning of the rest of your life. You are not at all the same person who went to bed a few hours before. Your body's cells have renewed themselves, and in the deep slumber of nocturnal meditation you have forgiven yourself for all the errors made the day before. You are fresh. Expect satisfaction of giving a sincere effort. Let your individual mind rest in the neutrality of the infinite mind.

THE ESSENTIAL PRACTICE

After the whole group has tuned in, there are six important parts to the core of sadhana.

Physical Preparation

This physical body is the temple of God. It allows us to manifest consciousness and move about on the material plane. It must be exercised to keep the circulation balanced and strong, to remove tensions and blocks created by emotions, to alter the glandular secretions so they correspond to the state of consciousness you want to attain, and to clean the blood system to prevent disease. With the best intentions and good thoughts, it is difficult to do a sadhana when you are sick. Take care of this physical body each day.

A strong exercise series awakens your will. You must press through the minor pains of limbering and nerve strengthening. This inflow of will power helps you beam the mind and stay alert during meditation and chanting. The exercises you practice should be sets as taught by the Siri Singh Sahib or a series strictly following his guidelines. They should leave you with a feeling of greater energy flow, mellowness, alertness, and enthusiasm. Too much exercise can tax the body so much that you will feel drowsy and lack motivation. A very heavy exercise and cleansing sadhana should be done when there is plenty of time to relax afterwards. A few examples of such a series is included in the kriya section. A balanced series of exercises that works on breathing, nerves, glands and spine is perfect for sadhana.

Mantra

In every sadhana you must chant an ashtang bij mantra, the Adi Shakti Mantra or the Panj Shabad. It is only by chanting with a proper breath rhythm that you create the Laya effect of suspending yourself into the infinite. We practice the physical preparation to be able to better experience this state. Guru Nanak said:

When the hands and body
are covered with dirt,
Water can rinse them clean.
When the clothes are dirty
and smeared with soil,
Soap can remove the stain.
When the mind is polluted
by error and shame,
It can only be cleansed by
the love of the Name. *

The Nam is the main solvent for mental stains. This is very sensible. The breath rhythm gives you access to the subconscious as well as the conscious mind. When you chant these mantras, your mind is fixed on the infinite aspects of yourself. You do not relate to polarities. You go into a neutral condition needed for a successful cleaning of the fears and patterns in the subconscious self. If a negative thought or fear comes to you, let it come but be conscious of the rhythm of **Sa-Ta-Na-Ma** or **Sat Nam.** The thought does not get the standard resistance or reaction it usually gets when coming into consciousness, so it moves more into the center of your consciousness to provoke a reaction. The fear or thought lives on the energy you feed it by either positive or negative attention. By focusing on the infinite you appear neutral to it even if you become temporarily emotional. As no reaction is returned to it, since you are neutral, it becomes neutralized. If you choose instead to fight the thought, you merely give it energy by giving it identity. By the mantra, you confirm *your* identity as the infinite truth and universal existence. You mind may object so let yourself ride on the mantra beyond the mind. If you decide to love the thought and become entranced by it, you still give it identity. So to stop the continual production and maintenance of the dualities of consciousness, you must become neutral. This is ultimately achieved only through mantra, since sound is the basic creative potential of your being.

* "Jap Ji," *Peace Lagoon*, M.S.S. Sardarni Premka Kaur Khalsa.

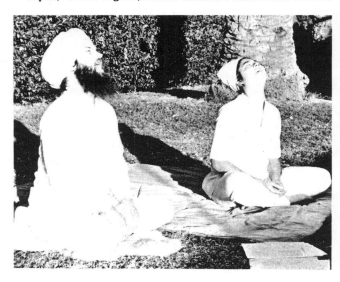

While there are many mantras Yogi Bhajan has taught that can be practiced as a part of your daily spiritual practices, we have a basic morning sadhana which Yogi Bhajan gave in 1992, to be practiced until the year 2013. It consists of seven parts and is described on pages 109-110 titled *Part I. Morning Sadhana for the Aquarian Age*. Models of sadhana for other times of the day are described in *Part II. Other Models of Sadhana* on pages 25-26.

Meditation

Doing mantra is a meditation. Any activity done in the right state of mind is a type of meditation, but here the reference is to silent meditation. It is that point in sadhana where you plunge into the total depths of the self with no outward stimulation to maintain you. This is where you test how well your inner being has awakened to support you. After every chant, take a few minutes to sit completely still without any movement and try to listen to the cosmic echo of the sounds you just produced. They are all around you, vibrating in the ether. If you can catch the subtle sound it will carry you without effort beyond the body consciousness into the sublime realms of self and bliss. It is for this that Guru Nanak said:

> By the hearing of God's Name
> Even the blind find their way.
> By the hearing of God's Name
> One grasps the infinite.
> O Nanak, the Devotee is
> Ever in bliss:
> By hearing the Lord's Name,
> His pain and sin are destroyed. *

After every exercise you should rest a minute and meditate to integrate the changes, experiences and sensitivity the exercise created. By practicing meditation after a kriya, you will be able to regain the state of consciousness produced by that kriya any time during the rest of the day by a few seconds of meditation.

Deep Relaxation

After exercises, chanting and meditation, you should deeply relax. The ability to relax is a divine quality. You are more centered within yourself and you become more sensitive to the energy patterns of your life. The effects of the kriyas and chanting are cumulative. They build for a long time after you have done them. Allow time for the energies you have released in the body and mind to circulate and come to equilibrium without involving your ego as a "director of the show." The energy knows where it should go; it is automatic. During relaxation you should cover your body with the meditation blanket or shawl so that you do not get cold. The amount of time you spend in deep relaxation depends on what you have done. Normally you should rest between 10 and 20 minutes. The state of consciousness you experience in this deep relaxation will not be just sleep. The glandular balance in the blood is altered, as is the functioning of the brain. You may have out-of-the-body experiences, you may have vivid dreams, you may remember nothing at all after closing your eyes. You will not, however, go into a regular shallow sleep unless you continue relaxing for an extended time. The best position for deep relaxation is corpse pose: lie on your back with your arms at the sides, palms up, ankles uncrossed and eyes closed.

Kirtan

After you journey through inner space, you must always reconnect with the world and daily duties. Sit with everyone and have a joyous song fest, singing the praises of the Infinite and the joys of life. Kirtan is an active singing rather than a deep meditation. It is the harmony of voices and instruments. It is realizing you are in a group of people who have purified themselves and are ready to actively live the day in truth and righteousness. Kirtan lets you reenter wordly consciousness but with a difference. You tend to remember the tunes throughout the day and with every breath, utter the Nam.

Prayer

Prayer is a potent capacity in man. Prayer is when the finite consciousness addresses the infinite self. Open your heart and be thankful for all the people who created and carried this consciouness through time so you could enjoy it now. You can ask for anything you want in prayer, for the Giver is infinite, and He gives all. If one's heart can open in compassionate prayer for humility, every heartbeat can bring a miracle.

In the Sikh tradition, we always offer the **Ardas which reminds us of our historical predecessors and our present duty to uphold consciousness and righteousness. A very universal way to offer a prayer is to dedicate part of your life force to what you pray for. Yogi Bhajan often gives an example of a prayer such as the following, which uses the breath:

> Inhale and hold your breath,
> For the peace of the world,
> For the health of all, to make everybody happy,
> So those who are lonely may have their partner,
> And God may find mercy on everybody,
>   on each individual.
> Say this prayer on this breath
> And please exhale.
> This is the charity of the breath.

** A copy of the English translation of this prayer may be found in the "Ardas," in *Psyche of the Soul* by Dr. Sant Singh Khalsa (1993).

* "Japji Sahib," *Peace Lagoon*, M.S.S. Sardarni Premka Kaur Khalsa.

Inhale again.
Pray for all dear ones,
   related ones, known, unknown,
   on the whole planet, for those
   who are sick, those who are unhappy,
   unhealthy or need spirit.
Send this thought by doing a prayer
   on this breath, let it go.
Inhale deep again to end all causes
   and effects which affect any man
   and make him unhappy,
   for anything that brings war
   and destruction,
   for anything which brings hatred
   and jealousy,
Say a prayer on this breath
   *and let it go. ***

The universality of prayer for self-guidance and humility is shown in this prayer given by the Siri Singh Sahib at the end of a class:

Oh Formless in every form,
Oh Infinite of every finite,
Oh Unknown, known through
   the entire creation,
Oh, Beyond, still bound by love,
It was Thy grace that you spoke
   and You heard,
You made it possible that all people,
Thy creatures, could come
   and could share Thy grace.
Give us power to walk
   on the path of righteousness;
Give us humility to serve
   and find love of our brother;
Give us tranquility and peace to find
   the higher realms of consciousness.
May Thy grace lead us
   to the light of infinity;
May our trip to the world be successful,
To spread Thy service so the
   fellow mankind can share.
May this day bring us a
   peaceful onward journey.
May Thy grace prevail,
And may You lift us
   to the levitated consciousness.
Oh God of Gods, oh Lord of Lords,
   if you have been so kind and merciful
   to bring us together with Thee,
   oh Infinite, oh Unknown, oh Beyond
   still bound by love.
Give us the power of happiness,
   joy and bliss, so we can live
   in the ecstasy of consciousness.
                              *Sat Nam. ***

* UCLA Advanced Class; Guru Ram Das Ashram,
Los Angeles 3/26/74.

23

SADHANA AS A METATHERAPY

Sadhana is a soothing balm for the tensions of modern civilization. The pressures and rapid technological development of this century have radically changed the way people live. Our lifestyle in the megalopolis induces a split from nature's rhythms and consequently from the natural attunement to our inner life. This leaves a split that runs between the two sides of our Western brain. It is a popular notion to recognize that our brain has two sides which have differentiated functions. The same difference has been recorded by the yogis. The two sides deal with action, emotion, and perception in opposite ways. The chart below outlines the different functions attributed to the two sides by psychologists.

Qualities Attributed
To the Hemispheres of the Brain

LEFT HEMISPHERE	RIGHT HEMISPHERE
Logical or Analytical	Synthetic Perceptual (Intuitional)
Discrete	Diffuse
Verbal	Non-verbal
Propositional	Appositional
Numerical	Geometrical
Successive	Simultaneous

The West has pressed the left brain to the limit. We have filled our lives with action-oriented, goal-oriented, linear, logical, verbal thinking. The right brain that rules intuition and is the doorway to the deeper self has not been valued. But the right brain activities are equally as important as the left, and we have an innate drive to use all parts of ourselves. The frustrated right brain leads us to great gullibility in emotional and spiritual endeavors as we thirst for experience and leap at every opportunity. Since our left brain predominates we are usually interested in quick attainment, flashy experience, complex philosophy, secret cults, or rituals that give security through judgmental attitudes. Sadhana is a way of healing the left/right split and imbalance of our consciousness. It becomes a kind of therapy. Since it heals by stimulating the integrative mechanisms without the individual having to go into the origin of specific conflicts, it functions as a *meta*therapy.

In sadhana, the exercises and concentration are left hemisphere functions. The meditation and devotional chanting are right-brained. *Pratyahar* is a left-brain process but *Laya* is a right-brain activity. The exercises stimulate what the yogis call the central brain, ruled by the pituitary and pineal glands. Done every day, these exercises are not aimed at flashy experiences but gradually awaken the roots of the self.

Another element in the sadhana process is commitment. The Siri Singh Sahib once said that 90% of today's insanity comes from a lack of commitment and the capacity to commit. Commitments set the values of the self. The values of the self allow you to subject the power of the self to create. Creativity allows detachment. Detachment allows judgment. Judgment plus forgiveness give progress in the process of expansion of the self.

Sadhana acts as a counselor to the two sides of the self. It encourages a central self to become bilingual and translate the languages of the two sides. It creates a meditative mind which can absorb all the stimuli in the environment, compute it, and then act wisely instead of just reacting. The inner observer can understand logic as well as intuition, activity as well as rest, science as well as art. We must develop the bilingual self fully prepared with a clean sense of values and a deep capacity for commitment. This capacity comes through sadhana.

WAKE-UP EXERCISES

Before you wake in the morning your mind always gives you a signal to awake. At that signal, turn on your back with your eyes closed. Make your hands like cups and place them over your eyes. Look into the palms and slowly raise your hands to 1½ feet. Then stretch the legs forward, the arms over your head, and stretch like a cat. Arch the spine and flex all of your muscles both left and right. Then bring the feet together and raise them six inches from the ground, keeping the legs straight. Raise your head six inches and fix your eyes on your toes. Point your fingertips toward the toes with the arms beside the hips but not touching them. Hold this position for 1 to 3 minutes with long deep breaths or breath of fire. Relax for 2 to 3 minutes. Then bring the knees up to the chest and hold them to eliminate gas. Rock back and forth to massage the spine. Then sit up and come into easy pose with the arms straight and the hands in gyan mudra on the knees. Take at least 26 long, deep, complete breaths. Feel that energy is charging the bloodstream and the breath is recharging every cell in your body. Then, to build your aura, put your arms at sixty-degree angles from the horizontal with the fingertips on the pads of the hands. Do rapid nostril breathing (breath of fire) for 1 to 3 minutes. Inhale and bring your thumb tips together over your head. Then exhale and *feel great!*

MODELS OF SADHANA

The Models of Sadhana section is in two parts:

Part I.
Morning Sadhana for the Aquarian Age

This is the morning sadhana given by Yogi Bhajan in 1992 to be practiced until the year 2013. It is described in detail on pages 109-110.

A number of beautiful examples of this sadhana are available as audio tapes and CD's. For ordering information, you may contact your local 3HO or Kundalini Yoga Center or any of the following:

Golden Temple Enterprises
tel 505-753-0563; fax 505-753-5603

Ancient Healing Ways Catalog
tel 800-359-2940 in US or
tel 505-747-2860 outside the US;
fax 505-747-2868

Satnam Versand
Frankfurt, Germany
tel 069/43 44 19; fax 069/43 85 71

Part II.
Other Models of Sadhana

These are to be practiced at other times of the day, and are presented on pages 25-26.

PART II. OTHER MODELS OF SADHANA

For the years 1992 through 2013, Yogi Bhajan has designated a specific early morning sadhana. The following sadhanas can be practiced at any other time of day, while the *Sadhana for the Aquarian Age* is the early morning sadhana.

Model I is a good model of a 2-1/2 hour sadhana for the serious practitioner. It includes all aspects of a good sadhana.

MODEL I

A) Wake-up routine and preparation.

B) Optional reading of the Banis or chanting of an appropriate mantra to Guru Ram Das.

C) Entire group chants **Ong Namo Guru Dev Namo** three to five times.

D) Exercise 30 to 45 minutes.

1) Begin with 5 to 10 minutes of limbering exercises to thoroughly wake up and stimulate circulation. Emphasize stretching the life nerves and the spine. Exercises such as frog pose, cat-cow, spinal flexes, leg stretches or running in place are a few good examples.

2) Pranayam for 10 minutes. The teacher should guide this carefully.

3) A physical exercise kriya for 25 to 30 minutes.

4) Deep relaxation for 5 to 10 minutes.

5) Come out of the relaxation by rotating the wrists and ankles; then rapidly rub the palms of the hands and the soles of the feet together. Cat stretch four or five times, left and right. Pull the knees to the chest and rock back and forth to massage the length of the spine.

E) Chant any of the following for approximately one hour:

1) The 2-1/2 breath cycle **Ek Ong Kar Sat Nam Siri Whahe Guru**. Minimum time for this is 37-1/2 minutes.

2) The Panj Shabad **Sa-Ta-Na-Ma** for 31 minutes. Follow this with a total of 31 minutes of chanting the 2½ breath cycle **Ek Ong Kar,** and the Sarab Shakti Mantra: **Gobinday, Mukanday. . .** etc.

3) The Laya yoga form of **Ek Ong Kar Sat Nam Siri Wha Guru** for 31 minutes, followed by 10 minutes of the long **Sat Nam.**

F) Immediately after chanting sit silently. Meditate on the sounds which have been projected for 5 to 10 minutes.

G) Deep relaxation for 10 minutes. Come out of relaxation as in "D5" above.

H) Special or guided meditation for 5-31 minutes.

I) Chant **Guru Guru Wahe Guru, Guru Ram Das Guru** long enough to contact the divine energy.

J) Grace of God meditation for 10 minutes. (This may be done at another time.)

K) Kirtan as time permits.

L) Ardas and hukam.

MODEL II

A-C) Same as Model I.

D) Same as Model I , 2 through 5 only. Begin with a powerful cleansing pranayam for 15 to 20 minutes.

E-G) Same as Model I.

H) Vigorous exercise for 10 minutes, followed by a 15 minute meditation.

I-L) Same as Model I.

MODEL III.

A-C) Same as Model I.

D) Begin with 15 to 30 minutes of exercise as in Model I; then do a kriya that optimally is 31 minutes in length. This kriya should be practiced only 7 to 11 minutes at first. Repeat it each day and gradually increase the time towards mastery. Follow the kriya with 10 minutes of silent meditation. At this time you may choose another kriya to be repeated each day, gradually increasing the time to mastery, or you may choose to practice a different one each day to become familiar with other kriyas. This kriya should be done for only about 15 minutes. Again, meditate for 5 to 10 minutes. End this section of sadhana with 10 to 15 minutes of moderate exercise in which all the limbs have a chance to move. Prepare to sit for chanting.

E-G) Same as Model I.

H) This has already been included in "D" of this model.

I-L) Same as Model I.

MODEL IV.

This is a model for those times when you practice a 2½ hour sadhana of chanting the Nam. This should be done at least twice a year by every student-teacher. The 2½ breath cycle of **Ek Ong Kar** should be done one of these times. If possible, the other time should be reading from the *Siri Guru Granth Sahib*; otherwise, chant the **Ek Ong Kar** mantra again.

A-C) Same as Model I.
 D) Exercises for 20 to 30 minutes that are powerful but do not require a long relaxation, and prepare you to sit.
 E) Chant for 2½ hours in beautiful sonorous tones.
 F) Meditate silently on the sound for 5 minutes.
 G) Relax for 15 minutes.
 H) Excluded.
 I-L) Same as Model I.

VARIATION: Sometimes it is impossible to do the 2½ hours of chanting all in the morning. It is permissible to split it into two parts; in this case it is best to chant 1½ hours in the morning and the evening.

MODEL V

There are times when you need to practice deep silent meditation on the Nam. The prime hour for this is between 2:30 and 3:30 a.m., the calmest time of the day. The inner sound current is loudest at this time. A simple alteration of the schedule to accommodate this follows.

A-C) Same as Model I.
 D) Meditate 45 minutes to 1 hour.
 E) Exercise kriya 45 minutes to 1 hour.
 F) Chant 1 hour.
 G) Deep relaxation.
 H) Kirtan.
 I) Reading of the Ardas, and receiving a Hukam.

MODEL VI

This is an example of how you might start building a morning practice if you have had little experience and you want to increase your time commitment slowly.

A-C) Same as Model I.
 D) Choose three short exercise sets (20 minutes each). Alternate these sets in a three-day pattern so that no muscles become too sore and each part of your system gets a thorough workout.

 E) Rest for 5-10 minutes.
 F) Chant the Adi Shakti Mantra for 30 minutes or select a meditation that fits your needs. This takes about one hour a day and will give you energy and balance. Change the kriyas you practice every few weeks. Increase the time, moving toward Model I. When you become accustomed to the yoga, try doing the same set and meditation for forty days.

QUESTIONS OFTEN ASKED ABOUT SADHANA

Question: Should I change the exercises and kriyas every day?

Answer: One part of the sadhana should stay constant long enough for you to master, or at least experience, the changes evoked by a single technique. Each kriya and mantra has its individuality. Their effects are not all the same although they all levitate you toward a cosmic consciousness.

You may want to practice a spectrum of the many things Siri Singh Sahib Bhai Sahib Harbhajan Singh Khalsa Yogiji has shared with us. But at some point, stop window shopping and commit considerable attention and effort to one thing. Learn to value the pricelessness of *one* kriya and all others will be understood in a clearer light.

There is a natural forty-day rhythm to habits in the body and mind. It takes about forty days of consistent practice to break a habit. To establish a new habit in action and in the subconscious takes about ninety days. It is good to take these biorhythms into account when designing the sadhana for long-term results.

At least twice a year each teacher should accomplish a forty-day, 2½ hour sadhana of either chanting the 2½ breath, Ek Ong Kar mantra, or reading from the Siri Guru Granth Sahib.

Question: Is teaching a class in sadhana the same as teaching a class outside the ashram?

Answer: No. There are differences. No matter where you teach a class of exercises, it will be 60 minutes or less, including a relaxation. But in sadhana, there is regular attendance which allows everyone to focus on a particular kriya and gradually increase the length of practice. In a class, you might chant long *"Sat Nam"* for 7 to 10 minutes; in sadhana you could build it up to 31 or 45 minutes. Another difference is the amount of talking that should be done. In an outside class, there is more need for inspiring, coaxing and explaining. Sadhana occurs in the quiet, ambrosial hours. We should speak only of the Infinite, and mostly we should listen to the Infinite.

Question: If I have to leave sadhana, what is the best way?

Answer: The same way you entered. Be aware of the presence of the teacher by bowing in your consciousness. Be quiet so nothing is disturbed. Choose a time to leave that is between kriyas and meditations. A sharp noise during a deep meditation is a shock to the total system. Do not come and go as you please, but as would please the highest teacher.

Question: Should I wake someone up who falls asleep in sadhana?

Answer: No. God should wake him. The experience of sadhana is between the individual and God. Do not interfere. You can inspire beforehand. If sleeping is a chronic habit, discuss it with the person at a convenient time, but do not abruptly wake someone. He may be at a different level of experience than you think. It is our intention, of course, to stay totally alert and awake.

Question: When I am sick, should I attend sadhana?

Answer: If you are going to be in bed all day with an extreme sickness, then no. If it is not extreme (this includes most menstrual periods), then attend sadhana and do what you can. If you cannot exercise or meditate well, then at least attempt to meditate. Afterwards, lie down and rest in sadhana while mentally listening to the shabad. This way you will get well faster and maintain the rhythm of a regular sadhana. It also eliminates the tendency to have minor morning illnesses to escape the self-discipline of a constant sadhana. In other words, participation in a group effort, and regularity of discipline are paramount, but do not be a fanatic to the point of aggravating a serious illness.

Question: When ashram residents get home very late should they sleep through the group sadhana then get up and do their own?

Answer: If at all possible, they should be in the group sadhana. If there is a service project done by the whole ashram which keeps everyone up late, you might start group sadhana slightly later than usual. If a few people have work (like a nightshift etc.) or are doing a pre-arranged service, then it would be tolerable. Under no condition are late movies, spontaneous night walks, entertainment, etc. excuses for not being in group sadhana. We must remember to make morning sadhana a high priority and a cornerstone of our lifestyle.

Question: Can I do an individual sadhana?

Answer: It is fine anytime in the day that does not interfere with your commitments. That period of time before group sadhana begins is excellent. If you have a special health sadhana that you must do as assigned as yogic therapy by your teacher then you can do that. The general rule, however, is that individual sadhana is not a substitute for group sadhana. A prime goal of sadhana is to develop the group consciousness into a universal consciousness.

Question: I am a beginner and can only spend one hour on sadhana. Will one hour have any effect?

Answer: Always do some sadhana no matter how short, for every effort of the individual mind to meet the universal self is reciprocated a thousand-fold. The ideal is a perfect 2½ hour sadhana. But if we are to run, we must first learn to walk. An hour is excellent (see Model IV). As you grow into sadhana, you will find time to extend it if you really want to do so. It is good for some people to start more slowly. If you try to climb Mt. Everest without climbing even a foothill beforehand, failure could discourage you from all other attempts. Build slowly and constantly at a pace you can maintain, but definitely do *something*.

Question: As the leader of sadhana, should I participate in all the exercises?

Answer: As a leader, your responsibility is to set a good example and to give clear instructions for each step of the sadhana. You should do as many exercises as you can without becoming unaware of the group. You must check to make sure that everyone is doing the exercise properly before beginning yourself. Sometimes it will be better not to participate at all. Always join in during chanting. When teaching a class outside of sadhana, you should participate as little as possible in the physical exercise. Concentrate only on inspiring and serving the class members.

Question: When chanting in the morning, the pitch often gets low. What, if anything, should be done to change the pitch?

Answer: Chant at a constant, mid-range pitch as much as possible. If your breath rhythm is not correct, or your spine is not kept straight, or you do not take complete breaths in the Adi Shakti Mantra, the chant will lose energy and drop in pitch. If you project the sound of the mantra from the back of the mouth in a full and roundish way, the power of the chant will increase as you continue and the pitch will stay constant.

If you are constant and listen to the sound of your chant, you will hear different pitches. These are actually overtones of the basic sound you are creating. The overtones will be high-pitched, subtle and seem to float around the room. You cannot identify that tone with one person since it is formed by the combination of group sounds. The overtone is a good sign that the sadhana group is tuned in to each other and beyond each other. As you listen to the first overtone and become very calm, you may begin to hear even higher and more subtle overtones. This awareness aids meditation on the etheric echo of your chanting as you sit silently after chanting aloud.

If your group is in a unitive consciousness, no one will shift the pitch. If the pitch does shift, it will seem to do so by itself. It will shift smoothly and infrequently.

Question: Is it alright to harmonize with the main tone?

Answer: Chanting is not singing. It is vibrating all the cells of the body, all the thoughts of the mind and the core crystal of the soul to the same shabad. Chanting in meditation is beyond personality.

Chanting like a choir with many harmonies turns the group consciousness, which is striving for universality, into individual consciousness responding to social consciousness. Leave vocal harmonizing for kirtan and group song fests. Learn to harmonize the body, mind, and soul while chanting.

Question: Is it mandatory for the same person to lead sadhana every morning?

Answer: In all Kundalini yoga ashrams, the same teacher teaches every sadhana — Guru Ram Das. The individual who helps direct the sadhana is often the leader of the ashram. It is not necessary that it always be the head of the ashram. If other students are qualified to teach and can lead a good sadhana, it might be very beneficial for the group to experience the effects of slightly different styles of leadership.

Question: Are there different sadhanas for different days of the week?

Answer: Each day of the week has its own energy. In astrology this is symbolized by associating each day with a planet. (*See the chart on page 29 for all the qualities.*) The daily sadhana exercise series could be chosen to relate to these energies. An emotional, calming pranayam for Monday, a nabhi (navel point) kriya for Tuesday, a brain cleansing set for Wednesday, a deep meditation Thursday, a sex transmutation series Friday, a strenuous physical cleansing kriya Saturday, and a blissful projective laya yoga meditation Sunday. This is a good idea, but if you are varying the sadhana exercise daily, you will also find that each day of the week differs from week to week. Ultimately you must use your own sensitivity to choose what kind of energy to deal with in the exercises. If you have no strong feelings to the contrary, the chart may be used as a guide.

Question: Should I bring my children to sadhana?

Answer: Your children are the future. The future will only be as secure as the foundation that is built into the young generation. It is very inspirational to see the radiance from young children who attend the last portion of sadhana during chanting. Usually the young ones do not attend during exercises although very young ones may sleep through them and there is no restriction.

Whether or not your particular child should attend is an individual determination. If he has been raised in the yogic tradition where chanting and exercise are a natural part of his environment, then bring him. If he is very disruptive during sadhana, then his attendance should be discussed with the ashram family for a final decision.

Question: Is it important to wear a head covering?

Answer: During sadhana, be sure to cover your head with a non-static, natural cloth like cotton, and keep the hair up. The hair regulates the inflow of sun energy into the body system. To let the solar energy flow without obstruction, let the hair grow to its full natural length and take good care of it. If this is done, the amount of energy that goes downward from the seventh chakra increases tremendously. The kundalini energy is activated by the radiant force of the solar plexus and moves upward in response to the solar energy coming down. This balances the body energy and maintains the total equilibrium.

If the hair is down, unkept or uncovered so that it is electrically imbalanced, this natural process of raising the kundalini energy will be impeded.

Every major spiritual tradition has covered the head, but reasons often get lost through the centuries.

Question: Do we need a special place for sadhana?

Answer: In the ashram or your residence a special place or altar is ideal. The care you give the external environment is a sign and symbol to the mind of your intention. The outer reflects the inner. If the place of meditation is sloppy it usually means you do not value relating to that infinite self, or you value it but do not believe in it or yourself. When traveling you do your best to bring the sense of specialness with you to wherever you meditate. Some people use a portable meditation picture or incense to help induce this feeling.

DAY	PLANET	SYMBOL	QUALITY
Monday	Moon	☽	Emotional
Tuesday	Mars	♂	Energetic, combative
Wednesday	Mercury	☿	Business Communication
Thursday	Jupiter	♃	Expansion and Deep thought
·Friday	Venus	♀	Love, Sensuality
·Saturday	Saturn	♄	Karma, Constriction, Discipline
Sunday	Sun	☉	Purity, Energy of self

BASICS

Before beginning a set or meditation always sit in easy pose, put your hands together at the sternum in prayer pose and chant **Ong Namo Guru Dev Namo** at least three times (see Adi Mantra in the mantra section). This sequence will ready your mind to expand unto the Infinite.

If you are teaching Kundalini yoga, remember that students should experience no more than one hour of actual practice per class.

There are some breathing exercises (*pranayama*), postures (*asanas*), hand positions (*mudras*), sound currents (*mantra*), and body locks (*bandha*), which are used again and again in the practice of Kundalini yoga. Become familiar with these basics by reading this section thoroughly and experiencing each pranayam, asana, mudra, and mantra. In this way, when you begin to practice the exercise sets, these common actions will be familiar to you.

SOME BASIC BREATHING TECHNIQUES

Kundalini yoga employs a wide range of breathing techniques. They are more extensive and sophisticated than in any other form of yoga. The breath, its rhythm, and its depth are correlated to different states of health, consciousness, and emotion. Kundalini yoga uses the breath scientifically to change the states of energy. There are a few basic breaths that should be mastered in order to freely practice the kriyas.

DEEP BREATHING

The simplest of all the yogic breaths is just long deep breathing, but it is a habit that we, as a culture, do not have. Our normal tendency is to breath irregularly and shallowly. This leads to a totally emotional approach to life, chronic tension, and weak nerves. The lungs are the largest organ of the human body. The average lungs can enlarge to a volume of almost 6,000 cubic centimeters. Besides supplying oxygen to and removing carbon dioxide from the body, the respiratory system helps regulate body pH (acidity - alkalinity) and helps excrete water vapor, hydrogen and small amounts of methane. Normally we may use only 600 or 700 cubic centimeters of that capacity. If you do not expand the lungs to their full capacity the small air sacks in the lungs, called alveoli, cannot clean their mucous lining properly. Therefore you do not get enough oxygen and toxic irritants that lead to infections and disease build-up.

To take a full yogic breath you inhale by first relaxing the abdomen. Next expand the chest. As you exhale let the chest deflate first, then pull the belly in completely. The diaphragm drops down to expand the lungs and contracts up to expel the air.

By taking a deep yogic breath you can expand the lungs by about eight times. If you establish a habit of breathing long, deep, and slowly you will have endurance and patience. If you can take the breath down below eight times per minute the pituitary starts secreting fully. If the breath is less than four times per minute the pineal gland starts functioning fully and deep meditation is automatic.

BREATH OF FIRE

This breath is used consistently throughout the Kundalini Yoga kriyas. It is very important that breath of fire be practiced and mastered by the student. In breath of fire, the focus of energy is at the navel point. The breath is fairly rapid (2 to 3 breaths per second), continuous and powerful with no pause between the inhale and exhale. As you inhale, use the forward thrust of the nave point to bring the air into the lungs. As you exhale, the air is pushed out by pulling the navel point and abdomen towards the spine. In this motion, the chest area is moderately relaxed. This is a very balanced breath with no emphasis on either the inhale or exhale, and with equal power given to both.

Breath of fire is a cleansing breath which cleans the blood and releases old toxins from the lungs, mucous lining, blood vessels, and cells. Regular practice expands the lungs quickly. You can start with three minutes of breath of fire and build to twenty. Begin alternating three minutes of breath of fire with two minutes of rest for five complete sets.

SITALI PRANAYAM

This breath is often used to regulate fevers and blood pressure and to cure digestive ailments. To breathe this way just curl the tongue and extend the tip just past the lips. Inhale deeply, drawing the breath in the mouth through the curled tongue. Exhale through the nose. (See Sitali Kriya, page 79.)

BROKEN BREATHS

There is a wide range of broken breaths used in the kriyas. In these the inhale and exhale are divided into sections in specific ratios. Each ratio gives a different effect. Some typical ratios for inhale, hold, exhale, hold, are as follows: (1:4:2:0), (4:16:2:0), (4:0:1:0), and (1:8:1:8). As an example, examine the 4:1 ratio. This breath is used to heal oneself and to break depressions. You break the inhale into four equal sections. Each part is a quick sniff-like inhale that causes the sides of the nose to collapse in slightly. Exhale in a single breath through the nose. It is important to focus on the flow of the breath and to keep the broken breath equally divided.

WHISTLE BREATHS

In this type of pranayam you make a small hole

---

*For more detailed information of *breath of fire*, see *Summer Solstice Issue, 1975.* Kundalini Research Institute: Pomona, 1975.

between the lips by making a "pucker." Inhale and make a high-pitched whistle, then exhale through the nose. Another variation is to inhale through the nose and exhale with a whistle through the lips. Listen to the high-pitched sound as you breathe. This breathing changes the circulation and activates the higher glands such as the thyroid and parathyroid.

There are many other types of breathing but these are the basic elements of most breaths you will encounter.

ASANAS
BASIC SITTING POSTURES

Each exercise of a Kundalini kriya specifies what position to take. Sometimes the instruction for the sitting posture in the exercise or meditation is not fixed. The requirement may be to sit in any meditative or cross-legged pose, or to sit in an easy pose. In these cases the main requirement is for the spine to be straight and the posture to be balanced. Any of the sitting positions listed here would fit the requirements.

When you sit for meditation it is important that you feel balanced and stable. If you are leaning to one side or have great pain from the knees or ankles, you cannot meditate. If you do get into meditation in an off-balance posture you run the risk of misdirecting the energy and blood circulation that is stimulated by the kriya. Meditating in a chair, for example, is perfectly alright for those kriyas that allow it, but if you sit with the legs half dangling or with uneven pressure on the feet, then the blood distribution in the pelvis area will be imbalanced with respect to the two sides of the body. This in turn can offset the navel point which can lead to headaches, menstrual irregularity, digestive problems, and a host of minor pains that are difficult to find a cause for.*

Remember that the parts of the body are all interconnected and affect each other. Your posture should always feel well-balanced and comfortable to you. It should reflect harmony. In certain deep meditations your consciousness may alter to the degree that you temporarily lose your normal body awareness. In that case the posture must be balanced in such a way that is easy for the body to hold automatically without your conscious effort. If you are imbalanced then the muscles may jerk or spasm to adjust for stress. That little spasm can slightly rotate or displace a vertebra. When yoga was still new to this country, some entrepreneurs introduced meditation while doing the headstand. This was showy and tantalizingly different, but it led to many twisted necks and ruined meditations. With this in mind, choose any of the postures below and be conscious to set yourself well.

The surface you sit on must not be cold or too hard. That is why most yoga practitioners sit on a sheepskin or mat. A thick pad or large pillow doesn't work well because there is not enough support to stabilize the spine. A sheepskin is just the right thickness. It also provides an electromagnetic insulation from the ground. This prevents you from feeling tired or drained of energy as you meditate. The next best materials to sit on are wool, cotton, and silk. The worst surface to sit on is concrete or stone. Although you are designed with a natural pillow to sit on you still need to care for the spinal balance and electromagnetic integration of your nervous system.

LOTUS POSE

Sit with the legs extended forward. Spread the legs. Bend the left leg so the left heel comes to the groin. Lift the left foot onto the upper right thigh. Bend the right leg so that the right foot goes over the left thigh as close to the abdomen as possible. Straighten the spine. Lift the chest and press the lower spine slightly forward. This position will feel "locked in place." Once you are in it you can meditate very deeply and the position will maintain itself. There are very few exercises or meditations which require this posture, but it is recognized as one of the best asanas for deep meditation.

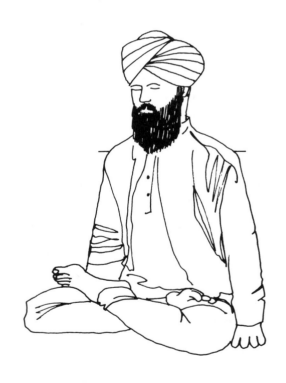

*Refer to the KRI Journal for the Study of Science and Consciousness, June, 1975 for a complete analysis of the effects of navel displacement and the yogic therapy approach to correcting such imbalances.

SUKASANA OR EASY POSE

There are three variations of sukasana which are commonly used in the exercises and meditations.

Variation Number One

Sit with the legs out straight. Pull the left foot in to the groin. Place the right foot over the ankle of the left foot so that it rests near the thigh. Straighten the spine. The feet can be arranged in either order.

Variation Number Two

A delicate and effective variation is to assume sukasana and then lift the heel of the foot near the groin. Come away from the body two or three inches. Arrange the foot on top so it rests directly on the calf with the ankle of the top foot about two inches up from the ankle of the bottom foot. In this pose make sure to press the lower spine forward. It will have a tendency to slip backward.

Variation Number Three

If the first two postures are too strenuous for you then try this variation. Sit up with both legs straight. Put one foot under the opposite knee and then draw the extended foot under the other knee. Pull the spine up straight and press the lower spine slightly forward.

All of these poses require less flexibility and are easier on the knees than the lotus pose. The drawback is that you must be more conscious of keeping the lower spine slightly forward so the upper spine can stay straight.

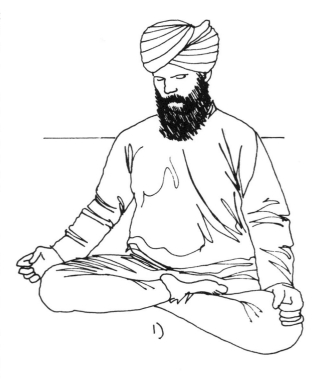

1)

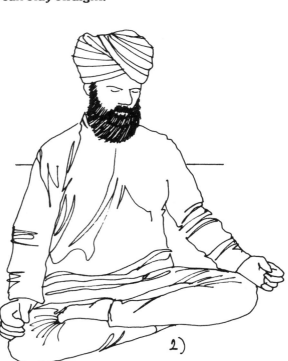

2)

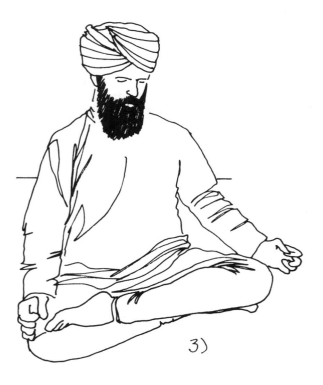

3)

32

SIDDHASANA (PERFECT POSE)

This posture is excellent for stimulating the nervous system and utilizing the body's sexual energy. It requires practice to perfect but once it is mastered simply sitting in this posture puts you into meditation.

Extend both legs straight. Bend the right leg and put the toes of the right foot in back of the left knee. Next bring the left heel under the right leg and under the sex organ. The left heel should touch the spot on the pelvis between the sex organ and the rectum. The toes of the right foot are contained in the bend of the left knee. Only the big toe is exposed. Pull the spine straight.

When you first begin to practice this asana do it for a few minutes only, building up gradually to as long as you like.

VAJRASANA (ROCK POSE)

This asana is well known for its beneficial effects on the digestive system. It gained its nickname from the idea that one who masters this posture can sit in it and "digest rocks." It also makes you solid and balanced as a rock.

To get in the position start by kneeling on both knees with the top of the feet on the ground. Sit back on the heels. The heels will press the two nerves that run into the lower center of each buttock. Keep the spine pulled straight.

HALF LOTUS

There are two poses frequently referred to as the half-lotus position. The easier one is a variation of sukasana. Sit in sukasana. Pull the top foot all the way across onto the upper thigh instead of leaving it near the ankle.

The other half lotus is a little more difficult. Sit in Vajrasana and then stretch the right leg out straight. Bend the right leg so the foot rests on the upper left thigh. You are sitting and balancing on the left heel and the right knee. The pose is sometimes done with the legs switched when specifically indicated.

SITTING IN A CHAIR

If none of these poses is comfortable for your meditation, you may sit in a chair if you remember to choose the chair wisely. You will have a tendency to totally relax or slump in a chair. Be sure to counter this impulse by reminding yourself that you are sitting down to become relaxed and totally attentive. Pick a chair which gives you firm support. A large over-stuffed lounge chair may be uncomfortable for a long meditation. The back of the chair can give you support if it is straight. A common error is letting the legs hang loosely. It is essential that the feet be equally placed on the ground. The equal placement will assure that your lower spine and hips do not get out of balance.

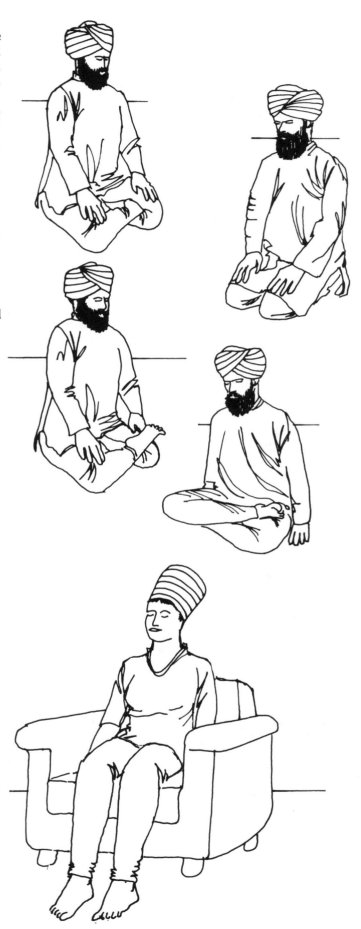

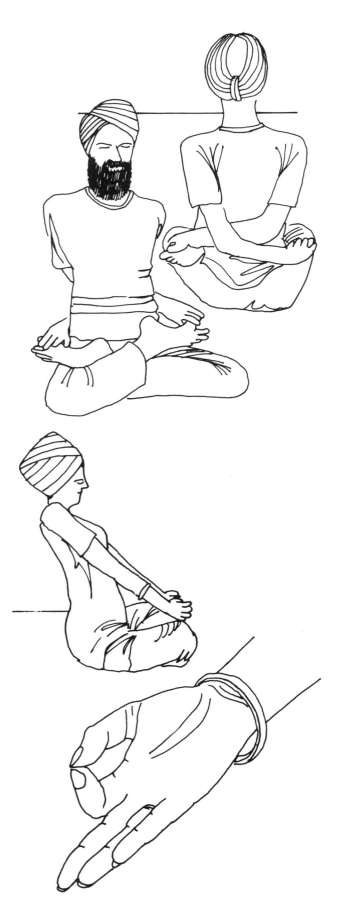

BOUND LOTUS

This posture is not as basic as the previous ones. It is difficult for many people. If you can do it, it is an excellent asana for deep meditation and glandular balancing. Get into the full lotus position. Push the feet as far up across the top of the thighs as possible. Reach around the back with both arms and grasp the toes. The right hand grasps the toes of the right foot. Similarly for the left hand and foot. Press the fleshy part of the big toes with the thumbs for pituitary stimulation. The spine is arched forward. The chin is held in. Do not force yourself into this position. Work slowly to gain the flexibility you need and begin to practice for a few minutes each day.

THIRTY-DEGREE SLANT

Sit in easy pose or lotus pose. Lean back 30° from the vertical but keep the spine straight. Don't slump back. Tilt the spine straight. This will create a small pressure at the third and fourth lumbar vertebrae. The eyes are usually open slightly for meditation in this pose. If you should suddenly relax, the spine would just bend backward in a natural manner.

BASIC MUDRAS

The hand is magical as well as functional. Early in life we use our hands in our first exploration of the world as we learn to manipulate it and create in it. The hand expresses our moods in each minute gesture. If you look at the palm you will see that the lines form intriguing patterns. If you understand the coding, the hands are an energy map of our consciousness and health. The yogis mapped out the hand areas and their associated reflexes. Each area of the hand reflexes to a certain area of the body or brain. Each area also represents different emotions or behaviors. By curling, crossing, stretching, and touching fingers to other fingers and areas we can effectively talk to the body and mind. The hands become a keyboard for input to our mind/body computer. Each mudra listed below is a technique for giving clear messages to the mind/body energy system.

GYAN MUDRA

To form gyan mudra put the tip of the thumb together with the tip of the index finger. This stimulates your knowledge and ability. The energy of the index finger is often symbolized by Jupiter, the planet representing expansion. This mudra is the one most commonly used. It gives you receptivity and calmness. In the practice of powerful pranayams or exercises the "active" form of the mudra is often used. In this case you bend the index finger under the thumb so the fingernail is on the second joint of the thumb.

SHUNI MUDRA

To form shuni mudra place the tip of the middle finger on the tip of the thumb. This mudra is said to give patience and discernment. The middle finger is often symbolized by the planet Saturn. Saturn represents the task master, the law of karma, the taking of responsibility and courage to hold to duty.

SURYA OR RAVI MUDRA

This mudra is formed by placing the tip of the ring finger on the tip of the thumb. Practicing it gives revitalizing energy, nervous strength, and good health. The quality of the ring finger is symbolized by the sun or Uranus. The sun represents energy, health, and sexuality. Uranus stands for nervous strength, intuition and change.

BUDDHI MUDRA

To form buddhi mudra place the tip of the little finger on the tip of the thumb. Practicing this opens the capacity to communicate clearly and intuitively. It also stimulates psychic development. The little finger is symbolized by Mercury for quickness and the mental powers of communication.

VENUS LOCK

This mudra is used frequently in exercises. It derives the name because it connects the positive and negative sides of the Venus mound on each hand to the thumbs. The thumbs represent the ego. The Venus mound is the fleshy area at the base of the thumb. It is symbolized by the planet Venus which is associated with the energy of sensuality and sexuality. The mudra channelizes the sexual energy and promotes glandular balance. It also brings the ability to focus or concentrate easily if you rest it in your lap while in a meditative posture. To form the mudra place the palms facing each other. Interlace the fingers with the left little finger on the bottom. Put the left thumb tip just above the base of the thumb on the webbing between the thumb and index finger. The tip of the right thumb presses the fleshy mound at the base of the left thumb. Thumb positions are reversed for women.

PRAYER MUDRA

For this the palms of the hands are flat together. The positive side of the body (right, or male) and negative (left, or female) are neutralized. This is always used when initially centering yourself in preparation for doing a kriya.

BEAR GRIP

For bear grip place the left palm facing out from the chest with the thumb down. Place the palm of the right hand facing the chest. Bring the fingers together. Curl the fingers of both hands so the hands form a fist. This mudra is used to stimulate the heart and to intensify concentration.

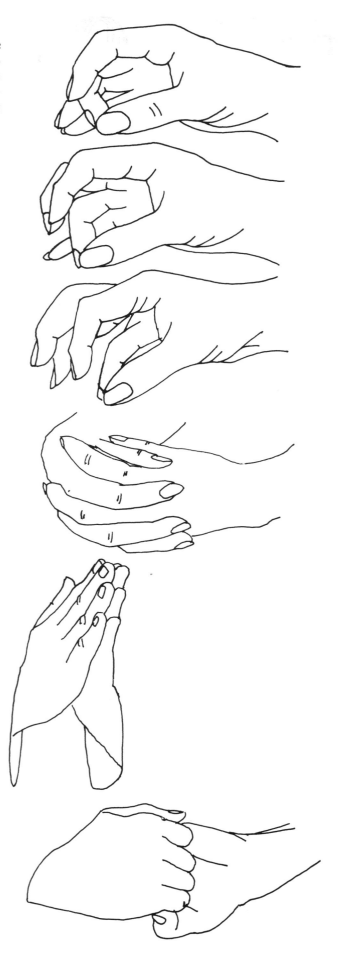

HANDS IN LAP

Another common mudra for meditation is formed by resting the left palm face-up in the lap with the right hand palm-up on top of it. Put the thumb tips together. The hand positions are reversed for a woman.

MANTRA

Mantra means mind projection: it is a technical device for regulating the mind. There are many mantras, each one having its own qualities, rhythm, and effects. The combined sound, resonance and rhythm of the mantra produce an altered state of consciousness which sets the pattern for the flow of thoughts. Mantra is not just an arbitrary label. It is a sound current which relates to its object. We always distinguish between a thing and its name because labels are arbitrary. Some languages make use of another level of sound. When a sound's innate vibration corresponds to or in some way reproduces what it refers to, it is a sacred language. This is the principle underlying languages such as Sanskrit and Gurmukhi. Chanting these ancient syllables is the fastest possible vibratory union between ourselves and the Creator. The mantra decides to which level of consciousness you want to relate. The power of the mantra is decided by the level of consciousness you have. Mantra yoga is the technique of yoking the individual with the whole. It is accomplished by merging the sound of the unit consciousness with the universal consciousness through the rhythmic power of the mantra.

Mantra words projected toward infinity relate to that frequency. If your total orientation and vibration is to make a lot of money, words will reflect it. Chanting is the specialized use of one's vibratory capacities, taking the individual from his current position or level of development or standard of living to his estimated or projected destination. Mantra is the principle of reinforcement and of rehearsal for the attainment of that ultimate destination.

In Mantra yoga not only do we categorize the sounds according to their effects, but also according to their effectiveness and level from which they originate. *Bakri* refers to the sounds made at the tip of the tongue. It is audible sound. It is what you speak. *Khanth* is the sound generated at the throat. It is the sound of the mind, the thinking sounds. Practically speaking, it is the sound which one forms mentally when reading silently, where you hear the subvocal sound as though actually physically projected. *Hardhay* is the sound formed at the heart center. It is the communication generated from the heart. It is the wish the mother sends to her son or the chela (disciple) sends to the guru. It is a communion via the silent language of thought. *Nabhi* refers to the sound formed at the navel. What we speak at the navel is most powerful. The last category is *Anhatha*, the sound which has no end, infinite. It is the "unstruck sound," which reverberates deep into all levels of consciousness and existence.

In the deepest meditation when the mind and body merge in union with the spirit essence, Anhatha is the sound that is heard. This anhad, or vibratory sound current is actually heard in children and its highest conscious development occurs around the age of one and one-half years. In modern society, with all the cluttering of our consciousness that industrialized society produces, this sound, which should otherwise be easily and regularly experienced, gradually loses its prominence in the mind and is usually unheard and forgotten by the age of three. It is through the practice of mantra and the remembrance of the name and sound of creative infinity that one may revitalize and redevelop that lost potential.

All these levels of sound are developed and integrated in a good sadhana over a long period of time. Ultimately the practice of mantra is perfected so that all mantra is *japa. Ja* means sound, *pa* means resound. *Japa* means "to resound the mantra." In japa the mantra is projected to the infinite cosmos and reflected back to you. You can hear it without feeling you produced it. It is the experience of a million voices echoing the mantra. It is cozy and creative. This japa leads to *tapa,* the inner psychic heat of prana. It is *tapa* that cleans and strengthens the nerves. The practice of japa is often done with the aid of a string of beads known as a *mala.* A mala is designed with a calculated number of beads (usually 108, 54 or 27). On each bead the mantra or meditation is repeated. In addition there is a "guru bead" or *meru,* which is slightly larger than the rest and remind the practitioner that he has completed one full cycle of the mala. The guru bead is not crossed, one merely turns the mala on it and returns in the direction he started from. Originally the mala was used to measure the length of time of the meditation practiced. Instead of doing a meditation for, say, thirty-one minutes, one might "do twenty-five malas." In addition, the necessity of changing direction every one-hundred and eight repetitions helps to maintain alertness, which may decline after many repetitions of the same mental sequence or mantra.

The mala also seems to provide a source of stimulation for the nervous system and brain through the continuous pressing of the fingertips on the beads. These are cut with crevices to minimize friction.

In all chants it is important to move the mouth. There is a tendency to mumble and make slurred mouth movements. The total effect of mantra depends on the reflex points on the tongue and in the mouth. So enunciate and move the tongue precisely.

I. ADI MANTRA: ONG NAMO GURU DEV NAMO

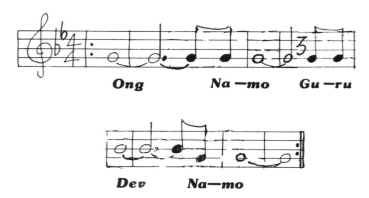

Ong   Na—mo   Gu—ru

Dev   Na—mo

This mantra is chanted before every class or practice session involving Kundalini yoga. If you read most old books about yoga, they say Kundalini yoga is the most powerful of all yogas, but that it is dangerous. The fact is that if you practice it in correct form, chant a universal Nam, and humble yourself before the higher self or teacher, it is perfectly safe. The Adi Mantra opens the protective channel of energy for Kundalini yoga.

Ong is the infinite creative energy experienced in manifestation and activity. It is a variation of the cosmic syllable *Om* which is used to denote God in His absolute or unmanifested state. When God creates and functions as Creator, He is called **Ong.**

Namo has the same root as the word *Nameste* which means "reverent greetings." *Nameste* is a common form of respectful greeting in India accompanied by the mudra of palms pressed together at the chest or forehead. It implies bowing down. Together **Ong Namo** means "I call on the infinite creative consciousness," opening yourself to the universal consciousness that guides all action.

Guru is the teacher or the embodiment of the wisdom that one is seeking. **Dev** means divine or of God, in a non-earthly, transparent sense. **Namo,** in closing the mantra, reaffirms the humble reverence of the devotee. Taken together, **Guru Dev Namo** means "I call on the divine wisdom," whereby you bow before your higher self to guide you in using the knowledge and energy given by the cosmic self. To chant this mantra you should be sitting with a straight spine, with the palms of the hands joined so that the joints of the thumbs are at the sternum. The mantra is usually chanted at least three times, with one and a half breaths per cycle with a full breath taken to begin and a half breath at the rest. Inhale and chant **Ong Namo**; inhale a half breath and chant **Guru Dev Namo.** The sound **Dev** is chanted a minor third interval higher than the other sounds. In musical notations if the other syllables were chanted at C, then **Dev** would be at D#.

II. ASHTANG AND BIJ MANTRAS

There are two types of mantras frequently used in Kundalini yoga. The first is the *bij* mantra, which is like a seed. It is the name of God planted inside of you, in your heart, where it will grow and spread its radiance throughout your total aura. But before the seed can be planted, the soil must be prepared. And for that we use an ashtang mantra. Ashtang means "eight-fold." Just as the spermatozoa must circle the egg eight times before penetrating, so too must the bij mantra be implanted in the heart within the eight-fold vibration of the ashtang mantra. The eight-fold vibration acts as a stimulant that balances the entire brain. It is only an ashtang mantra or the *Panj Shabad* mantra that can provide this total stimulation of your potential.

Adi Shakti Mantra:
EK ONG KAR SAT NAM SIRI WHAHE GURU

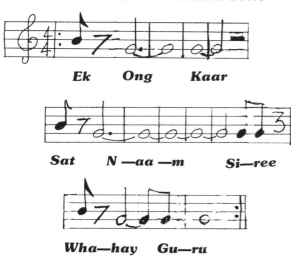

Ek   Ong   Kaar

Sat   N—aa—m   Si—ree

Wha—hay   Gu—ru

There are many ashtang mantras, but one that we chant most regularly is called the Adi Shakti Mantra.

There are two ways to find the Divine. One way is to open the solar plexus and charge your solar centers so that you get directly connected. The other method is to concentrate and meditate and get the sound of shabad within your solar centers so that you get the divine light. This mantra incorporates both methods.

The mantra is a precise sound: **Ek Ong Kar Sat Nam Siri Whahe Guru.** They are exact keys which you touch to telegraph your message to the infinite self. Your entire system is played by these sounds. Each sound vibrates and integrates a different chakra to its full radiance within the aura. **Ek** means one. It is the essence of all which is one. **Ong,** as stated above, is the primal vibration from which all creativity flows. You go beyond all limiting conceptions of the world, and self, and penetrate to the creative core that supports it all through the sound of **Ong.** The sound is created in the upper palate and nose. It vibrates the entire skull and has a full nasal tone. *Kar* means creation. *Sat* means truth; *Nam* means name. The name of the One Creator known through creation is not a word, but truth. When you chant *Sat*, briefly contract the navel and lower centers to release some of the inner power of creation. *Siri* means great. *Wahe* is the untranslatable expression of one experiencing the Creator's supreme power. It is ecstasy. Guru means the wisdom, the sense of higher wisdom. So the eight vibrations are *Ek Ong Kar Sat Nam Siri Wahe Guru*. It can translate as: "There exists one Creator throughout the creation whose name is truth. Greatest is the ecstasy of that supreme wisdom."

The mantra may be divided into three parts. *Ek Ong Kar* means, "There is one Creator who has created this creation." Here you realize the need for a conscious union with the infinite. *Sat Nam* means "Truth is His Name." *Sat Nam* is the name of God that we relate to; it is the bij mantra, the seed that we are planting in our hearts. With *Sat Nam*, we pierce to the core of truth and understand the nature of reality. The third part of the Adi Shakti Mantra is *Siri Wahe Guru*. It means "great, indescribable beyond words is His wisdom." Here you express the bliss of truly knowing yourself. As the Siri Singh Sahib has said, "If you chant this mantra during these dark ages of the Kali Yug, it will open the lock of ignorance and darkness. This will liberate you and unite you with the Divine. In the period of two and one-half hours before the rising of the sun, when the channels are most clear, if the mantra is sung in sweet harmony, you will be one with the Lord. This will open your solar plexus, which in turn will charge the solar center. The solar complex will get connected with the cosmic energy and you will be liberated from the cycles of karma that bind you to this earth. All mantras are good because they all awaken the divine, but this mantra is the mantra for this time. It represents the path of progressive spiritual knowledge of the self."

Chanting this mantra means unlimited attachment to the infinite beyond any man or finite form. Those who attach themselves to a man or personality end miserably. This brings union with the ultimate cosmic energy. The Siri Singh Sahib says, "It is equal to millions and billions of suns. When you will recite this mantra, the day shall come when you shall have the light within you. You will find it equal to you cannot say what. There is no vocabulary and there is no tongue which can just say how bright that light is. But remember that light you shall see. That is the only light through which you can overcome the cycle of karma. Then nothing disturbs you. Then you live normally, and you are beyond the power of the cycles of time and space."

There is no need for secret mantras and all the gimmickry so often resorted to. This mantra is open to all without initiations and cults, yet it is basic to awakening and regulating the Kundalini energy: the basic evolutionary force in the total human psyche. This mantra may be chanted in the two and one-half breath cycle for its full power, or in any tune you make up for light meditation. In the two and one-half breath cycle, you take a deep inhale and chant *Ek Ong Kar* in one breath. The *Ek* is very short, *Ong* and *Kar* are equal in length. Take another deep inhale and chant *Sat Nam Siri*. The *Sat* is short, *Nam* is very long, and *Siri* just escapes your tongue with the last bit of breath. Then take a short half breath and chant *Wahe Guru. Wha* is short and *Guru* is long.

Bij Mantra: SAT NAM

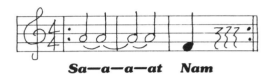

Sa—a—a—at   Nam

Sat Nam is the bij, or seed mantra that is most used in the practice of Kundalini yoga. It is a universal mantra which is not limited to Kundalini yoga. It represents the sound embodiment of Truth itself: *Sat* (truth), the reality of what exists; *Nam* (name, identity), the vibration which creates what it names.

When *Sat Nam* is chanted in its bij form, it is usually chanted in a breath ratio of 35 to 1 or 8 to 1. That is, the time of *Sat* is 8 or 35 times that of *Nam.* This mantra can be used to smooth out and balance mental energy. It gives you a feeling of reality. It can also be used to release energy.

As you chant this mantra extend your mind to Infinity and remember that in the beginning there was the word, and the word was God. This God, this word, lives inside of you. You are a manifestation of that. Tune into that Infinity. Project a call from your heart. The Infinity that created you is not deaf; and does not live very far away. The power of mantra is the power of manifestation. If we recite the mantra with the intensity of innocence, it will take the mind and heart to an experience of its origin in the Creator.

Continued next page.

Ashtang-Bij Mantra

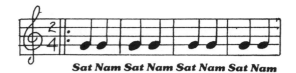

Sat Nam Sat Nam Sat Nam Sat Nam

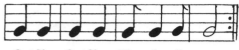

Sat Nam Sat Nam Wa — he Gu —ru

This is an ashtang mantra that uses only bij mantras as syllables. One of the most potent and frequently used mantras is **Sat Nam, Sat Nam, Sat Nam, Sat Nam, Sat Nam, Sat Nam, Wahe Guru.** This mantra works the tongue. Your throat will get dry at first until you master the rhythm. It can create the power of creative sound in your words. Each **Sat Nam** is one count in the rhythm. **Wahe Guru** is two counts. One repetition takes about 3 to 4 seconds. To keep the rhythm there is a slight inhale on a half-count between repetitions.

III. *PANJ SHABAD*: SAA-TAA-NAA-MAA

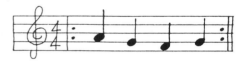

Saa Taa Naa Maa

This is the nuclear form of the bij mantra, **Sat Nam.** Here each syllable of sound is created in a ratio to the other. Adding this breath rhythm makes the mantra a form of Laya yoga. The five primal sounds are **SAA-TAA-NAA-MAA. SAA** means infinity; **TAA** life; **NAA** death; and **MAA,** rebirth or resurrection. The fifth sound is the common **AA,** which means "to come." These five sounds are known as the Panj Shabad.

IV. *SARAB SHAKTI MANTRA*: GOBINDAY, MUKANDAY, UDAARAY APAARAY, HAREEANG, KAREEANG, NIRNAAMAY, AKAAMAY

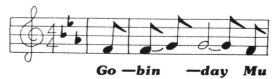

Go —bin —day Mu

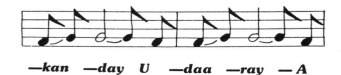

—kan —day U —daa —ray — A

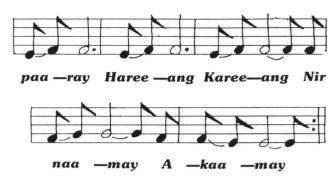

paa —ray Haree —ang Karee—ang Nir

naa —may A —kaa —may

This is a mantra with a very special quality: It eliminates karmic blocks and curses from the past, and cleanses the aura so that it becomes easier to meditate and relate to the Infinite. It was given by Guru Gobind Singh and is found in the tenth Guru's work, "Jaap Sahib." It is also an ashtang having eight major components. If this mantra is practiced regularly for 31 minutes to 2½ hours daily, it will cause all the occult powers to serve you. The mantra translates: "Sustainer, Liberator, Enlightener, Infinite, Destroyer, Creator, Nameless, Desireless." These are eight aspects or names of the Godhead. The mantra cleanses the subconscious and produces the shakti sun energy in every nerve. If a person is too mentally and physically blocked to let the vibratory effect of the Adi Shakti Mantra take hold, this mantra will clear the way. It is chanted in the above musical notation, with one full cycle per breath.

V. *GURU MANTRA*: GURU GURU WAHE GURU, GURU RAM DAS GURU

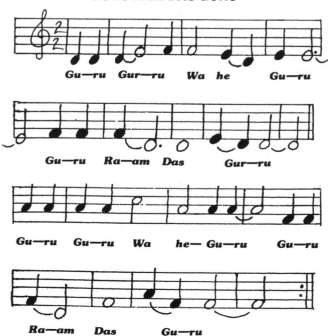

Gu—ru Gur—ru Wa he Gu —ru

Gu —ru Ra—am Das Gur —ru

Gu—ru Gu—ru Wa he— Gu —ru Gu—ru

Ra—am Das Gur—ru

This mantra relates directly to healing and protective energy represented by Guru Ram Das, the fourth guru of the Sikhs. He is held in reverence by all people who respect universal service. It is by the grace of the house of Guru Ram Das that through his channel, Siri Singh Sahib Bhai Sahib Harbhajan Singh Khalsa Yogiji, the veils of secrecy have been lifted from the teachings of Kundalini yoga. This mantra is an ashtang mantra. It was given to the Siri Singh Sahib from a deep meditation on Guru Ram Das, his guru on the etheric plane. It is comprised of two parts. The first part is a *nirgun* mantra (**Guru Guru Wahe Guru**). The second part is a *sirgun* mantra (**Guru Ram Das Guru**). *Nirgun* means without quality. A nirgun mantra is one which vibrates only to infinity, having no actual finite components. A *sirgun* mantra is one which represents form. This guru mantra projects the mind to infinity, then allows a finite guiding relationship to come into your practical activities. The first part of the mantra, **Guru Guru Wahe Guru**, projects the mind to the source of knowledge and ecstasy. The second part, **Guru Ram Das Guru**, means "the wisdom that comes as a servant of the infinite." It is the mantra of humility. It reconnects the experience of infinity to the finite.

The mantra is chanted a number of ways: the most common one is given in musical notation above. Try to complete full cycles of the mantra with each breath. It will give you relaxation, self-healing and emotional relief.

VI. *MANTRA OF ECSTASY:* WHA-HE GURU

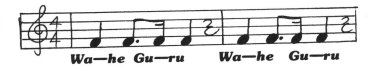

Wa—he Gu—ru   Wa—he Gu—ru

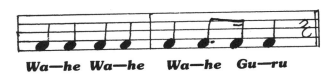

Wa—he Wa—he   Wa—he Gu—ru

The bij mantra, **Wa-he guru**, done in an ashtang form is *Wahe Guru Wahe Guru Wahe Wahe Wahe Guru.* It is a mantra that produces a sense of happiness. It is often used in kriyas that develop healing abilities. It has a rhythm that is the Laya yoga form so it easily stays with the subconscious with minimal practice.

There are many other mantras, but this collection has most of the basic chants needed for an excellent beginning to the practice of sadhana.

VII. *ADI SHAKTI MANTRA:* LAYA YOGA FORM

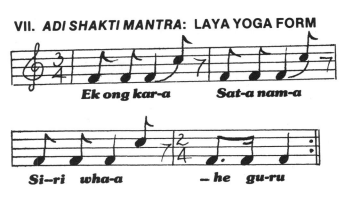

Ek ong kar-a   Sat-a nam-a

Si-ri wha-a   — he gu-ru

Besides the 2½-cycle chanting of the Adi Shakti Mantra there is a Laya yoga form which is very powerful and can suspend the mind into a kind of blissful trance of connectedness. The mantra is changed slightly by adding the "A" sound that we used in the Panj Shabad. This gives rhythm and extra power: **Ek Ong Kar-a, Sat-a Nam-a, Siri Wha-a, He Guru.** The rhythm of the chant gives it a sense of "spinning." It rotates the energy of all the chakras and the aura. The navel point is pulled in sharply on **Ek**. On each **a** (pronounced like *u* in *bus*) the diaphragm is pulled up so that the rib cage lifts. On **He** (sounds like *hay*), the stomach and diaphragm relax. As you chant, visualize the energy spinning from the base of the spine upward through the top of the head to infinity. With **Ek** see the energy start from the navel point and go downward. On the first **a**, the energy pierces the first chakra at the base of the spine. On the second **a**, it coils through the lock on the spine at the level of the diaphragm and heart center. On the third **a**, you spin the energy past the neck and throat chakra. On **He Guru** let the energy go through the top of the skull, the 7th chakra, into infinity. If you get into the rhythm of the spin, the breath will automatically ebb in and out at 2½ cycles per chant. The spine will heat up and sweat. It is a mantra of total absorption into infinity.

BASIC BODY LOCKS

There are certain combinations of muscle contractions that are called *bhandas* or locks. These are very frequently applied. Each lock has the function of changing blood circulation, nerve pressure, and the flow of cerebral spinal fluid. They also direct the flow of psychic energy, *prana*, into the main energy channels that relate to raising the kundalini energy. They concentrate the body's energy for use in consciousness and self-healing. There are three important locks: *jalandhara bhand*, *uddiyana bhand*, and *mul bhand*. When all three locks are applied simultaneously, it is called *maha bhand*, the great lock.

JALANDHARA BHAND

The most basic lock used in Kundalini Yoga is *jalandhara bhand*, the neck lock. This is practiced by sitting straight, lifting the chest and sternum upward, and gently stretching the back of the neck straight by pulling the chin back toward the neck. The head stays level without tilting forward. Straightening of the spine in the neck allows the increased flow of pranic energy to travel freely into the upper glandular centers of the brain. This is critical. In Kundalini Yoga kriyas, a vast energy is generated that produces psychic heat which opens the pranic *nadis* (channels) that may be blocked. When this blocking happens, there can sometimes be a quick shift in blood pressure causing dizziness; *jalandhara bhand* can prevent this phenomenon.

By applying this lock, the thyroid and para-thyroid glands get pressure that causes them to secrete optimally and activate the higher functions of the pituitary. If the lock is not applied, the breathing exercises can cause uncomfortable pressure in the eyes, ears, and heart.

It is a general rule to apply jalandhara bhand in all meditations unless otherwise specified.

UDDIYANA BHAND

This is the diaphragm lock. It is applied by lifting the diaphragm up high into the thorax and pulling the upper abdominal muscles back toward the spine. This creates a cavity that gives a gentle massage to the heart muscles. It is considered to be a powerful lock since it allows the pranic force to transform through the central nerve channel of the spine up into the neck region. It also has a direct link to stimulating the hypothalamic-pituitary-adrenal axis in the brain. It stimulates the sense of compassion and can give a new youthfulness to the entire body. The spine should be straight. It is normally applied on the exhale. Applied forcefully on the inhale, it can create pressure in the eyes and heart.

In Laya yoga, the rhythmic application of this lock is crucial to attaining the highest effects of chanting.

MUL BHAND

The root lock is the most complex of the locks and it is frequently applied. It coordinates and combines the energy of the rectum, sex organs, and navel point. *Mul* is the root, base, or source. The first part of the mul bhand is to contract the anal-sphincter and draw it in and up as if trying to hold back a bowel movement. Then draw up the sex organ so the urethral tract is contracted. Lastly, pull in the navel point by drawing back the lower abdomen towards the spine so the rectum and sex organs are drawn up toward the navel point. This action unites the two major energy flows of the body: prana and apana. Prana is the positive, generative energy of the upper body and heart center. Apana is the downward flow of eliminating energy. The root lock pulls the apana up and the prana down to the navel point. The combination of the energies generates the psychic heat that can release the kundalini energy. This lock is applied with the exhale. It is also applied on the inhale when specified.

MAHA BHAND

This is the application of all three locks at one time. When all the locks are applied, the nerves and glands are rejuvenated. The practice and perfection of maha bhand is said to relieve wet dreams and preoccupation with sexual fantasy. It regulates blood pressure, reduces menstrual cramping, and puts extra blood circulation into the lower glands: testes, ovaries, prostrate, cowper's glands, skene's glands, etc.

KRIYAS

A *Kriya* is a techniques used in Kundalini yoga to produce an altered state of consciousness.[*] This technique can be a meditation or an exercise or both.

Every exercise is not a kriya. By doing a kriya a sequence of physical and mental events are initiated that affect the body, mind and spirit simultaneously. Each kriya makes a specific claim as to its effect.

In this section you will find more than kriyas. These kriyas are of varying difficulty. Some, such as *Sat Kriya*, are a single exercise-meditation, while others are complete exercise sets followed by a particular meditation. Accompanying each kriya is a commentary on the physical, mental, and/or spiritual effects produced by practicing it. When a kriya is mastered, the practitioner gains "Easy and immediate access to a particular state of emotion or consciousness."[*]

All of the kriyas, as well as the information included in the sections on basics and meditation, are directly from the teachings of Siri Singh Sahib Bhai Sahib Harbhajan Singh Khalsa Yogiji, master of Kundalini yoga, the yoga of awareness.

[*] Gurucharan Singh Fowlis, "Kundalini Energy," *Kundalini Quarterly*, Fall Equinox, K.R.I. Publications, Pomona, California, 1976.

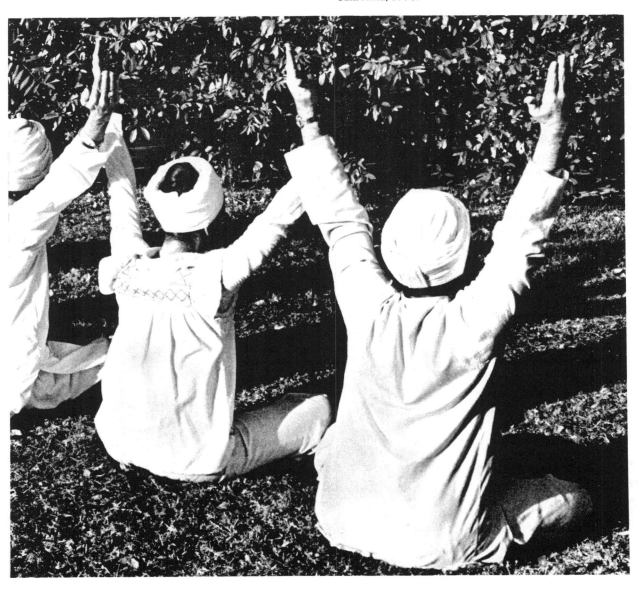

KRIYAS

SAT KRIYA

Sit on the heels and stretch the arms over the head so that the elbows hug the ears (A). Interlock all the fingers except the first ones (index) which point straight up (B). Begin to chant *"Sat Nam"* emphatically in a constant rhythm about eight times per 10 seconds. Chant the sound *"Sat"* from the navel point and solar plexus, and pull the umbilicus all the way in toward the spine. On *"Nam"* relax the belly. Continue at least 3 minutes, then inhale and squeeze the muscles tightly from the buttocks all the way up the back, past the shoulders. Mentally allow the energy to flow through the top of the skull. Ideally, you should relax for twice the length of time that the kriya was practiced.

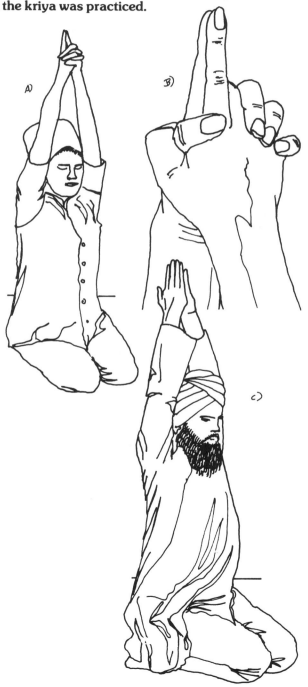

COMMENTS:

Sat Kriya is fundamental to Kundalini yoga and should be practiced every day for at least 3 minutes. Its effects are numerous. Sat Kriya strengthens the entire sexual system and stimulates its natural flow of energy. This relaxes phobias about sexuality. It allows you to control the insistent sexual impulse by rechannelizing sexual energy to creative and healing activities in the body. People who are severely maladjusted or who have mental problems benefit from this kriya since these disturbances are always connected with an imbalance in the energies of the lower three chakras. General physical health is improved since all the internal organs receive a gentle rhythmic massage from this exercise. The heart gets stronger from the rhythmic up-and-down of blood pressure you generate from the pumping motion of the navel point. This exercise works directly on stimulating and channelizing the kundalini energy, so it must always be practiced with the mantra *"Sat Nam."*

You may build the time of the kriya to 31 minutes, but remember to have a long, deep relaxation immediately afterwards. A good way to build the time up is to do the kriya for 3 minutes, then rest 2 minutes. Repeat this cycle until you have completed 15 minutes of Sat Kriya and 10 minutes of rest. Finish the required relaxation by resting an additional 15 - 20 minutes. Do not try to jump to 31 minutes because you feel you are strong, virile or happen to be a yoga teacher. Respect the inherent power of the technique. Let the kriya prepare the ground of your body properly to plant the seed of higher experience. It is not just an exercise, it is a kriya that works on all levels of your being—known and unknown. You might block the more subtle experiences of higher energies by pushing the physical body too much. You could have a huge rush of energy. You may have an experience of higher consciousness, but not be able to integrate the experience into your psyche. So prepare yourself with constancy, patience and moderation. The end result is assured.

If you have not taken drugs or have cleared your system of all their effects, you may choose to practice this kriya with the palms open, pressing flat against each other (C). This releases more energy than the other method. It is generally not taught this way in a public class because someone in the class may have totally weakened his nerves through drug abuse.

Notice that you emphasize pulling the navel point in. Don't try to apply mul bhand. Mul bhand happens automatically if the navel is pulled. Consequently, the hips and lumbar spine do not rotate or flex. Your spine stays straight and the only motion your arms make is a slight up-and-down stretch with each *"Sat Nam"* as your chest lifts.

If you have time for nothing else, make this kriya part of your every day promise to yourself to keep the body a clean and vital temple of God.

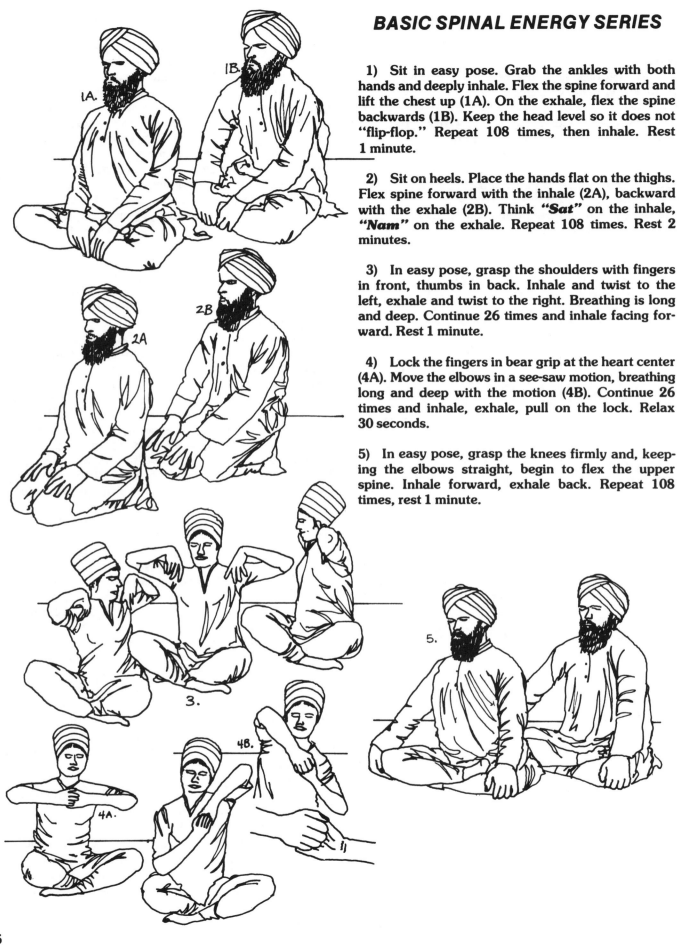

BASIC SPINAL ENERGY SERIES

1) Sit in easy pose. Grab the ankles with both hands and deeply inhale. Flex the spine forward and lift the chest up (1A). On the exhale, flex the spine backwards (1B). Keep the head level so it does not "flip-flop." Repeat 108 times, then inhale. Rest 1 minute.

2) Sit on heels. Place the hands flat on the thighs. Flex spine forward with the inhale (2A), backward with the exhale (2B). Think **"Sat"** on the inhale, **"Nam"** on the exhale. Repeat 108 times. Rest 2 minutes.

3) In easy pose, grasp the shoulders with fingers in front, thumbs in back. Inhale and twist to the left, exhale and twist to the right. Breathing is long and deep. Continue 26 times and inhale facing forward. Rest 1 minute.

4) Lock the fingers in bear grip at the heart center (4A). Move the elbows in a see-saw motion, breathing long and deep with the motion (4B). Continue 26 times and inhale, exhale, pull on the lock. Relax 30 seconds.

5) In easy pose, grasp the knees firmly and, keeping the elbows straight, begin to flex the upper spine. Inhale forward, exhale back. Repeat 108 times, rest 1 minute.

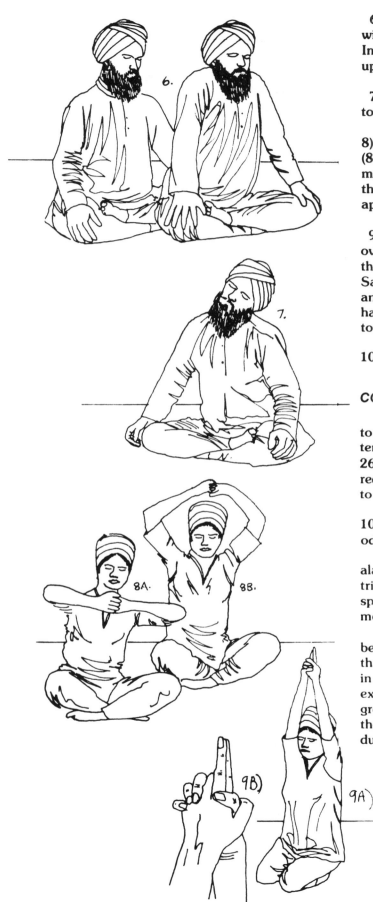

6) Shrug both shoulders up with the inhale, down with the exhale. Do this for less than 2 minutes. Inhale and hold 15 seconds with shoulders pressed up. Relax the shoulders.

7) Roll the neck slowly to the right 5 times, then to the left 5 times. Inhale, pull the neck straight.

8) Lock the fingers in bear grip at the throat level (8A). Inhale — apply mul bhand. Exhale — apply mul bhand. Then raise the hands above the top of the head (8B). Inhale — apply mul bhand. Exhale — apply mul bhand. Repeat the cycle two more times.

9) Sat Kriya: Sit on heels with arms stretched over the head (9A). Interlock the fingers except for the two index fingers which point straight up (9B). Say *"Sat"* and pull the navel point in; say *"Nam"* and relax it. Continue at least 3 minutes. Then inhale—squeeze the energy from the base of the spine to the top of the skull.

10) Relax completely on your back for 15 minutes.

COMMENTS:

Age is measured by the flexibility of the spine; to stay young, stay flexible. This series works systematically from the base of the spine to the top. All 26 vertebrae receive stimulation and all the chakras receive a burst of energy. This makes it a good series to do before meditaton.

In a beginner's class, each exercise that lists 108 repetitions can be done 26 times. The rest periods are then extended from 1 to 2 minutes.

Many people report greater mental clarity and alacrity after regular practice of this kriya. A contributing factor is the increased circulation of the spinal fluid, which is crucially linked to having a good memory.

A study done by Neil Goodman, Ph.D., December, 1973, at University of California at Davis, showed that the spinal flex exercise created large changes in EEG activity during and after the exercise. The exercise has a "multi-stage reaction pattern" that greatly alters the proportions and strengths of alpha, theta and delta waves. More research is being conducted.

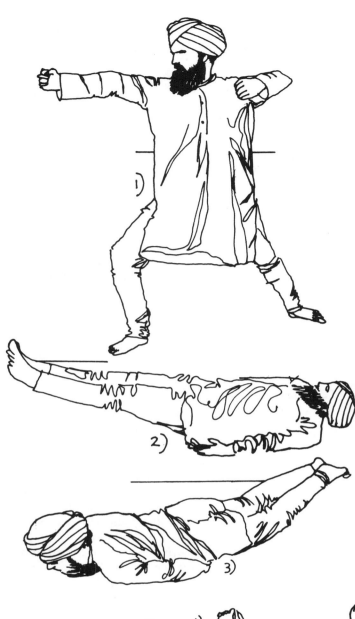

FLEXIBILITY AND THE SPINE

1) **Archer Pose:** Stand with the right leg bent forward so the knee is over the toes. The left leg is straight back with the foot flat on the ground, at a 45° angle to the front foot. Raise the right arm straight in front, parallel to the ground and make a fist as if grasping a bow. Pull the left arm back as if pulling the bowstring back to the shoulder. Feel a tension across the chest. Face forward and fix the eyes above the fist to the horizon. Hold the position 3 to 5 minutes, then switch legs and arms and repeat.

2) Immediately lie on the back. Put the heels together and lift both legs two feet from the ground. Hold the position 1 to 3 minutes with long deep breathing.

3) **Locust pose:** Lie down on the stomach. Make fists with the hands and put them on the lower abdomen inside the front hip bones near the groin. Keeping the heels together and the legs straight, lift them up as high as possible and hold this position for 3 minutes.

4) **Bow pose:** Still on the stomach, reach back and firmly grasp the ankles. Arch the back up from the ground and balance by pulling the ankles. Hold the position for 2 to 3 minutes.

5) Stand up straight and spread the legs two feet apart. Touch the right hand to the floor in front of the left foot. The left arm is pointing back. Switch sides and continue this alternate motion with long breaths. On the inhale, rise up completely; on the exhale touch the toe. Repeat 25 times on each side.

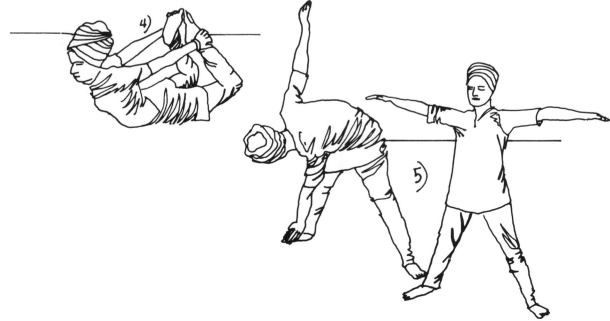

6) Stand up with the legs 6 inches apart. Bend forward and place the palms flat on the ground and exhale (6A). Inhale and rise up stretching backwards with the arms over the head (6B). Continue 25 times.

7) Stand with the legs 6 inches apart. Bend sideways stretching the arm over the head. Alternate smoothly from side to side, inhaling down and exhaling up. Do not let the body bend forward or backward. Continue 25 times on each side.

8) Sit down and extend the legs out in front, spreading them wide. Grab the big toe of each foot by locking the forefingers around the toe and the thumb pressing the toenail. Keeping a firm grip on both toes, inhale and arch the spine up straight. Exhale and touch the head to the right knee. Inhale to the original position, and exhale down to the left knee. Continue to alternate toe touches 25 times on each side. Inhale, hold the breath and exhale.

9) In this same sitting position, bring the legs together while still holding onto the toes. Inhale and arch up, exhale and pull the head down to the knees. Continue this pumping motion 25 times.

10) Plow pose: Lie flat on the back. Slowly raise the legs over the head until they touch the floor. The arms should be over the head pointing towards the toes. Keep the knees straight and point the toes towards the head, stretching the heels back. Relax in this position for 5 minutes. Slowly lower the legs back down to the ground.

Continued next page.

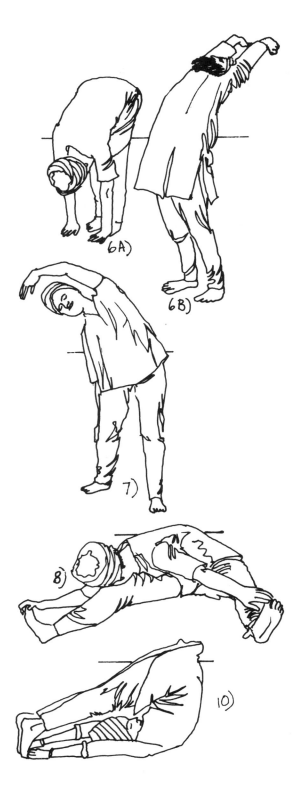

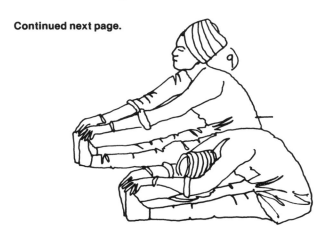

11) Shoulder stand: Come into this position by raising the legs straight up towards the ceiling (11A). Support the spine perpendicular to the ground with the hands. Let most of the weight be on the elbows. Hold this position for 3 to 5 minutes. Then bring the legs down in back of the head as in plow pose, but spread the legs wide apart (11B). Slowly go from this position to shoulder stand 4 times. Lower the legs and spine and rest on the back.

12) Come into plow pose with the arms along the ground in back of the spine (12A). Alternate from plow pose to lying flat on the back (12B). Continue 50 complete times. The hands may be used to lift the legs up and back. Relax for 3 minutes.

13) Sat Kriya: Sit on the heels with the arms overhead and the palms together. Chant "**Sat**" and pull the navel point in, chant "**Nam**" and release it. Continue powerfully with a steady rhythm for 5 minutes. Inhale, apply mul bandh and draw the energy up the spine to the brow point.

14) Immediately bend forward in *gurpranam*: Place the forehead on the ground and stretch the arms overhead, keeping the palms together. Meditate at the brow point by silently projecting the primal sounds, *"Sa Ta Na Ma."* Continue for 31 minutes.

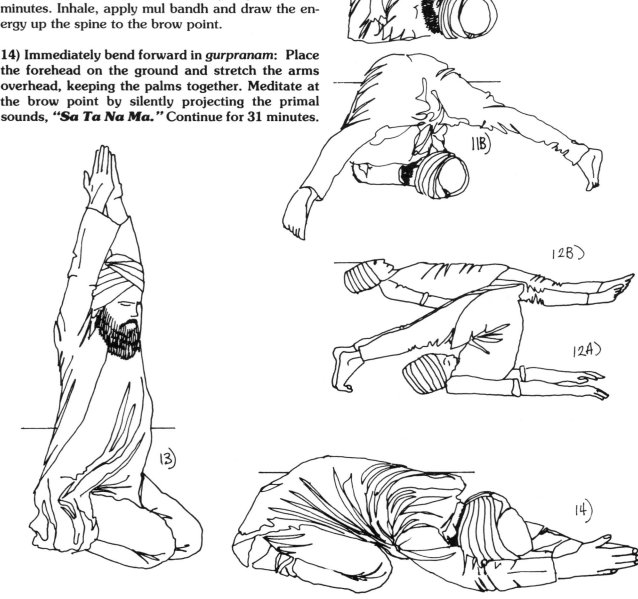

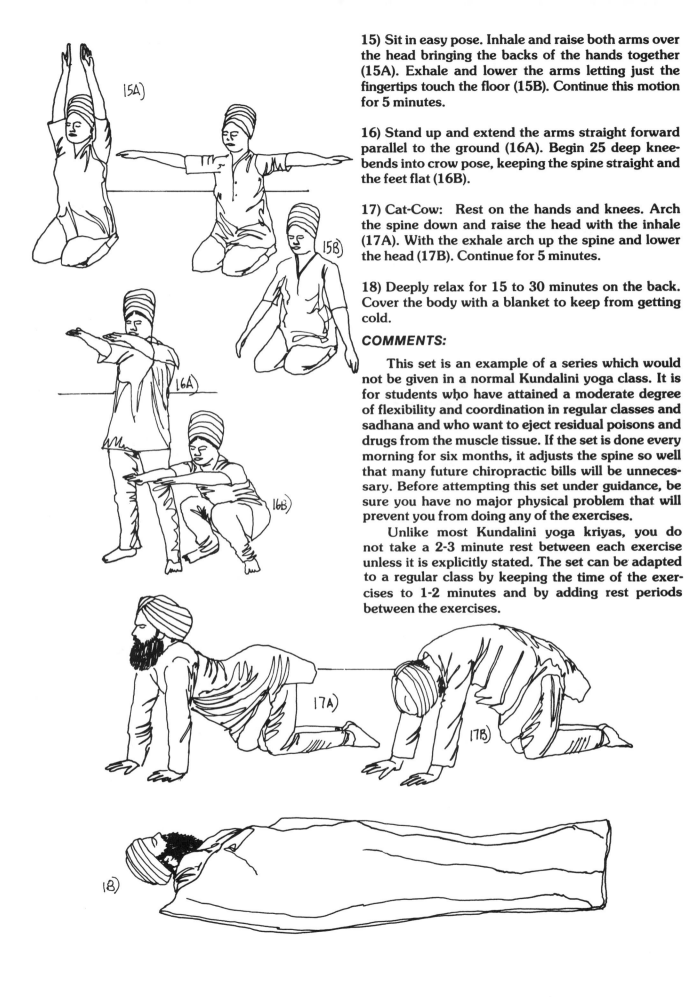

15) Sit in easy pose. Inhale and raise both arms over the head bringing the backs of the hands together (15A). Exhale and lower the arms letting just the fingertips touch the floor (15B). Continue this motion for 5 minutes.

16) Stand up and extend the arms straight forward parallel to the ground (16A). Begin 25 deep knee-bends into crow pose, keeping the spine straight and the feet flat (16B).

17) Cat-Cow: Rest on the hands and knees. Arch the spine down and raise the head with the inhale (17A). With the exhale arch up the spine and lower the head (17B). Continue for 5 minutes.

18) Deeply relax for 15 to 30 minutes on the back. Cover the body with a blanket to keep from getting cold.

COMMENTS:

This set is an example of a series which would not be given in a normal Kundalini yoga class. It is for students who have attained a moderate degree of flexibility and coordination in regular classes and sadhana and who want to eject residual poisons and drugs from the muscle tissue. If the set is done every morning for six months, it adjusts the spine so well that many future chiropractic bills will be unnecessary. Before attempting this set under guidance, be sure you have no major physical problem that will prevent you from doing any of the exercises.

Unlike most Kundalini yoga kriyas, you do not take a 2-3 minute rest between each exercise unless it is explicitly stated. The set can be adapted to a regular class by keeping the time of the exercises to 1-2 minutes and by adding rest periods between the exercises.

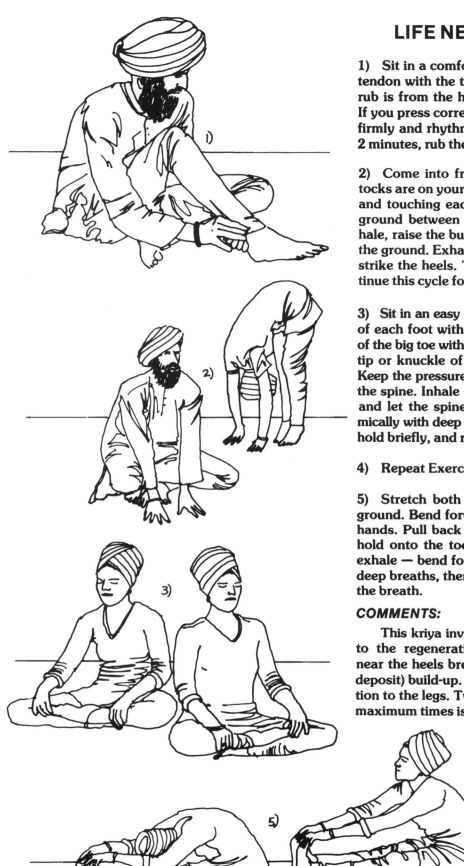

LIFE NERVE STIMULATION

1) Sit in a comfortable pose. Massage the Achilles tendon with the thumbs of both hands. The area to rub is from the heel up the tendon about 4 inches. If you press correctly, the toes will flex slightly. Rub firmly and rhythmically. After rubbing one foot for 2 minutes, rub the other foot for 2 more minutes.

2) Come into frog pose: Squat down so the buttocks are on your heels. The heels are off the ground and touching each other. Put the fingertips on the ground between the knees. Keep the head up. Inhale, raise the buttocks high, keeping the fingers on the ground. Exhale, come down and let the buttocks strike the heels. The exhale should be strong Continue this cycle for 3 to 5 minutes.

3) Sit in an easy cross-legged pose. Grasp the big toe of each foot with your hands. Press the fleshy part of the big toe with 10-15 lbs. pressure. Use the thumb tip or knuckle of the thumb to apply the pressure. Keep the pressure strong and constant. Begin to flex the spine. Inhale — press the spine forward. Exhale and let the spine flex backwards. Continue rhythmically with deep breaths for 3 minutes. Then inhale, hold briefly, and relax the breath.

4) Repeat Exercise 2 for 3 to 5 minutes.

5) Stretch both legs out straight in front on the ground. Bend forward and grasp the toes with both hands. Pull back on the toes for 30 seconds. Then hold onto the toes as you inhale — arch up, then exhale — bend forward. Do 26 of these pumps with deep breaths, then inhale — arch the head up. Relax the breath.

COMMENTS:

This kriya invigorates the heart and gives energy to the regenerative and sexual system. Rubbing near the heels breaks up long-term crystal (calcium deposit) build-up. This in turn helps improve circulation to the legs. Two complete cycles of this kriya at maximum times is a good workout.

KRIYA FOR LOWER SPINE AND ELIMINATION

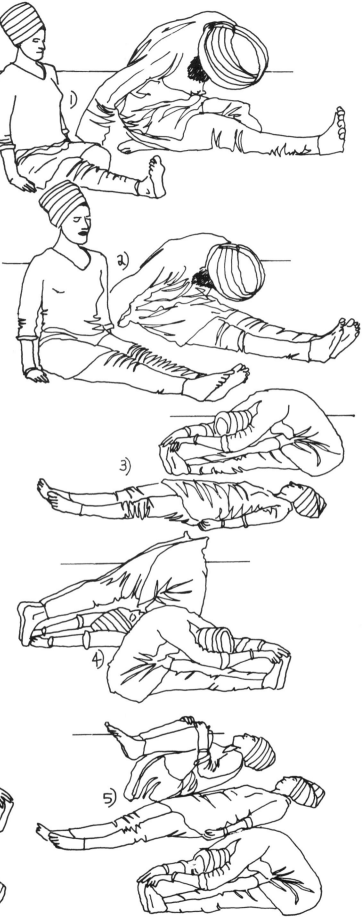

1) Sit up straight with the legs stretched out. Bring the left leg under the buttocks so you sit on the left heel. Place both hands palms down next to the hips. Inhale deeply. As you exhale bend forward. Inhale — raise up. Continue for 2 minutes.

2) Do the same as in Exercise 1 but keep both legs extended straight forward. Continue for 2 minutes.

3) Lie down on the back. Inhale deeply. As you exhale, sit up, grasp the toes, and bend forward. Inhale and lie down again. Mentally vibrate *"Sat"* on the inhale, *"Nam"* on the exhale. Continue with deep breaths for 2 minutes.

4) Lie on the back. Raise the legs slowly up until the feet touch the ground over the head. This is plow pose. Let the legs back down. Sit up and grasp the toes. Continue alternating between plow pose and the forward stretching smoothly and continuously for 2 minutes.

5) Lie on the back. Bring the knees onto the chest and press them close with your hands. Extend the legs straight on the ground. Sit up and grasp the toes. Continue this cycle rhythmically for 2 minutes.

6) Bend forward and grasp the toes with the legs out straight. Do not let go of the toes as you roll back on your spine until you are in plow pose. Roll back and forth without letting go of the toes. Continue for 2 minutes.

7) Relax completely.

COMMENTS:

The first, second and third chakras associated with the rectum, sex organs and navel point are thoroughly exercised in this kriya. It gives flexibility of the spine and improves the power of digestion and elimination of waste and toxins. It is not good to practice as a beginning set. You need some flexibility to do it well.

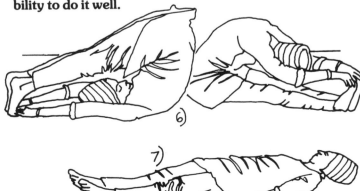

BEGINNERS CLEANSING SET

1) Lying on the back, place the hands in back of the neck in venus lock under any loose hair (1A & B). Begin breath of fire for 1½ minutes, inhale and hold for 20 seconds. Repeat breath of fire, inhale and hold for 30 seconds. Relax the breath. Inhale deeply raising both of the legs one foot high (1C). Hold for 15 seconds, exhale, inhale, and relax.

2) In this same position, spread the legs wide open. Begin breath of fire for 1 minute. Inhale — raise the legs 3 feet from the ground and hold for 5 seconds. Relax the legs on the ground. Repeat 3 times, doing breath of fire for 1 minute each time. Repeat breath of fire 1 more time, then inhale, raising the legs one foot. Hold as long as comfortable. This kriya stimulates the sex energy channels in the upper thigh.

3) Stretch pose: Lie on the back with legs together and raise the heels six inches. Raise the head and shoulders six inches and look at your toes. In this position begin breath of fire and continue for 3 minutes. Inhale and relax.

4) Sit up, with the legs out straight. Put the left leg on the thigh of the right leg. Keep the hands parallel to the ground, palms down, on each side of the left foot. Inhale, exhale and reach past the toes (4A). Inhale deeply and sit up leaning back 30° (4B). Exhale grabbing the toes. Repeat 25 times and switch legs.

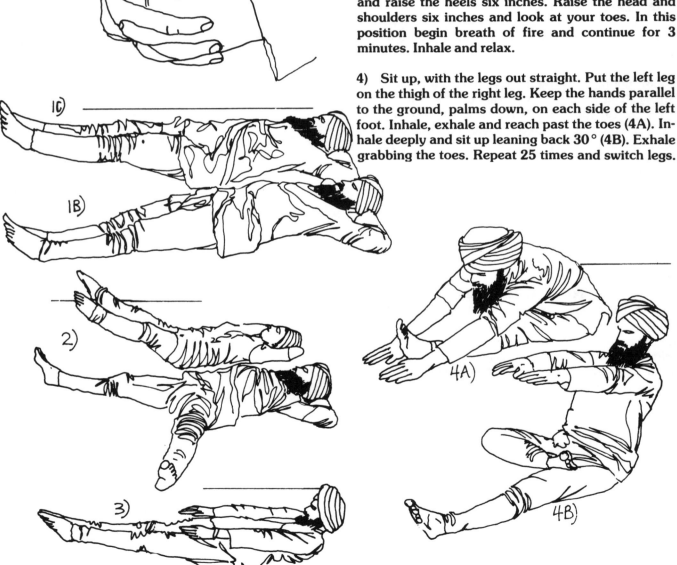

5) Sit up and lean back 60⁰ from the ground. Put the palms on the ground behind the back as a brace. Drop the neck back and look at the ceiling, fixing the eyesight on one point. Do not wink or blink. Begin breath of fire for 2 minutes. Inhale — raise both feet 12 inches from the ground, keeping the vision steady. Hold for 15 to 20 seconds, exhale down. Repeat breath of fire for 1 minute. Inhale — raise both feet 12 inches. Hold for 15 seconds. Exhale down and relax completely on the back.

6) Lying on the back, inhale deeply. Exhale completely. Raise hands to the sky, fingers outstretched (6A). Bring hands together into tight fists and slowly bring them down to the chest, bending elbows (6B). Keep tension in the arms as if struggling so that the fists shake as they touch the chest (6C). Relax the breath. Repeat the exercise with the breath held in. Deeply and completely relax for 5 minutes.

COMMENTS:

This easy series can beautify and lighten your body. Exercise 1 stimulates the navel point energy and blood circulation into the lungs. Exercise 2 adds the creative power of the sexual energy. Exercise 3 restimulates the navel point. Exercise 4 adjusts the chemical balance in the blood and helps the lower back and waistline. Exercise 5 moves the energy into the brain and eyes. It has helped cases of headaches and eye diseases such as cataract. Exercise 6 removes any residual tension and allows you to relax.

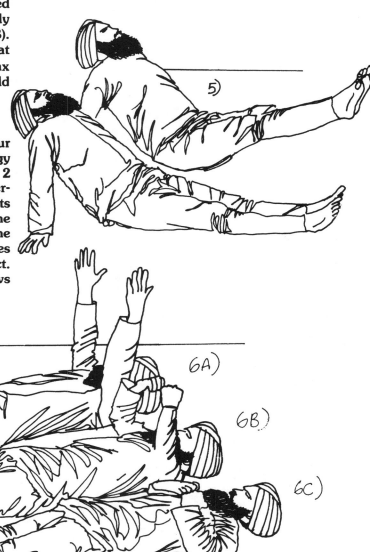

5)

6A)

6B)

6C)

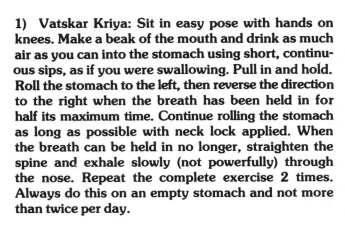

ELIMINATION (APANA) EXERCISES

1) **Vatskar Kriya:** Sit in easy pose with hands on knees. Make a beak of the mouth and drink as much air as you can into the stomach using short, continuous sips, as if you were swallowing. Pull in and hold. Roll the stomach to the left, then reverse the direction to the right when the breath has been held in for half its maximum time. Continue rolling the stomach as long as possible with neck lock applied. When the breath can be held in no longer, straighten the spine and exhale slowly (not powerfully) through the nose. Repeat the complete exercise 2 times. Always do this on an empty stomach and not more than twice per day.

2) Sit on the heels and touch the forehead to the ground. Keep hands down at sides. Imagine that there is a big tail coming off the end of the spine and wag it. Imagine the tail weighs 100 pounds and try to make it break the wall. Continue for 3 minutes followed by 5 minutes of rest.

3) Lie down on the back. Press the toes forward. Lift both legs three feet up. Start long deep breathing. Continue for 2 to 3 minutes. Inhale — hold briefly and relax.

4) Lying down on the back, bring the legs overhead and catch the toes. Roll back and forth from the base of the spine to the neck. Hold onto the toes and keep rocking for 3 minutes.

5) Sit up immediately in easy pose. As calmly as possible, make a "U" of the right hand and close the right nostril with the thumb of the right hand. Use the little finger to close the left nostril. Inhale

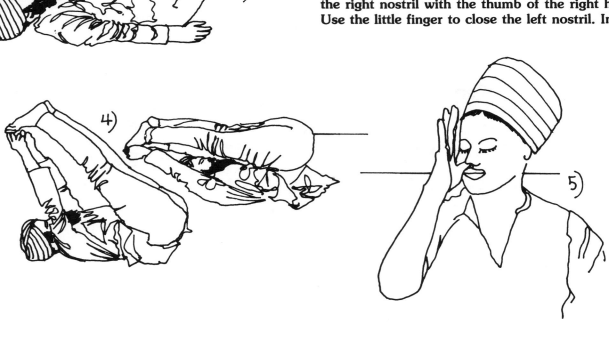

through the left nostril, exhale through the right. Continue for 3 minutes, then inhale and feel the energy radiate throughout the body, giving health and life.

6) Sit in easy pose. Interlace fingers and thumbs in front of the chest at the heart level with the palms facing the chest. Turn the head left and right. Inhale as the chin goes over the left shoulder, exhale as it turns right. Continue for 3 minutes.

7) Sit in easy pose, arms out parallel to the ground. Swing arms backward in a rolling motion as if swimming (7A). Continue for 1 minute. Inhale — bend the elbows to bring the fingertips onto the shoulders (7B). This remagnetizes the electric current. While the breath is held, the energy starts circulating. Exhale — let the energy flow to all parts and feel refreshed.

COMMENTS:

This is a good example of a simple but powerful series that was kept secret by those few yogis who learned it. This will allow you to completely master your digestive system and give a youthful appearance to your skin. Aging does not start with years; it begins with nutritional deficiency, intestinal problems, and an inflexible spine that disrupts the flow of spinal fluid.

Exercise 1 adjusts the acid-base balance in the stomach, but it must be done regularly without missing a single day. Exercise 2 strengthens the heart, Exercise 3 slims the waistline and cleans the gallbladder, Exercise 4 flushes the circulation and balances the nerves. Exercises 5 and 6 distribute the pranic force and stimulate the thyroid and parathyroid. Exercise 7 remagnetizes the aura.

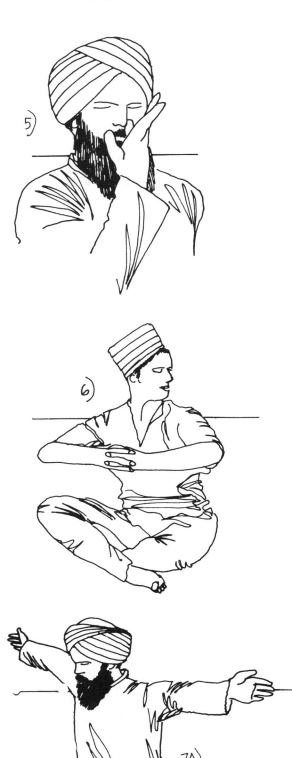

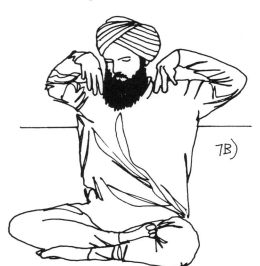

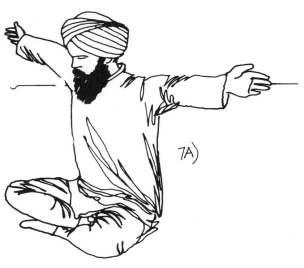

ABDOMINAL STRENGTHENING

1) Sit on the heels. Interlock the fingers (venus lock) behind the neck. Spread the elbows wide apart. Begin breath of fire for 2 minutes.

2) Lie on the stomach. Reach back and grab the ankles. Pull the ankles toward the buttocks keeping the chest on the ground. Hold for 2 minutes with normal breathing.

3) Stretch pose: Lie on the back. Raise the head and heels six inches off the ground. Point the hands toward the toes. Begin breath of fire for 2 minutes.

4) Lie on the back. Begin a bicycling motion with the legs keeping them parallel to the ground. Use deep breaths. Continue for 2 minutes.

5) Still on the back, keep the legs together with the toes pointed forward. Inhale and smoothly raise both legs to 90°. Then exhale as you lower them. Use deep breaths. Continue for 2 minutes.

6) Lie on the stomach. Place the palms on the ground under the shoulders (6A). Slowly arch up into cobra pose (6B). Lift the feet up toward the head (6C). Hold for 2 minutes.

7) Lie on the back. Bring both knees up to the chest and hold them there with the hands. Roll forward and back on the spine. Continue for 2 minutes.

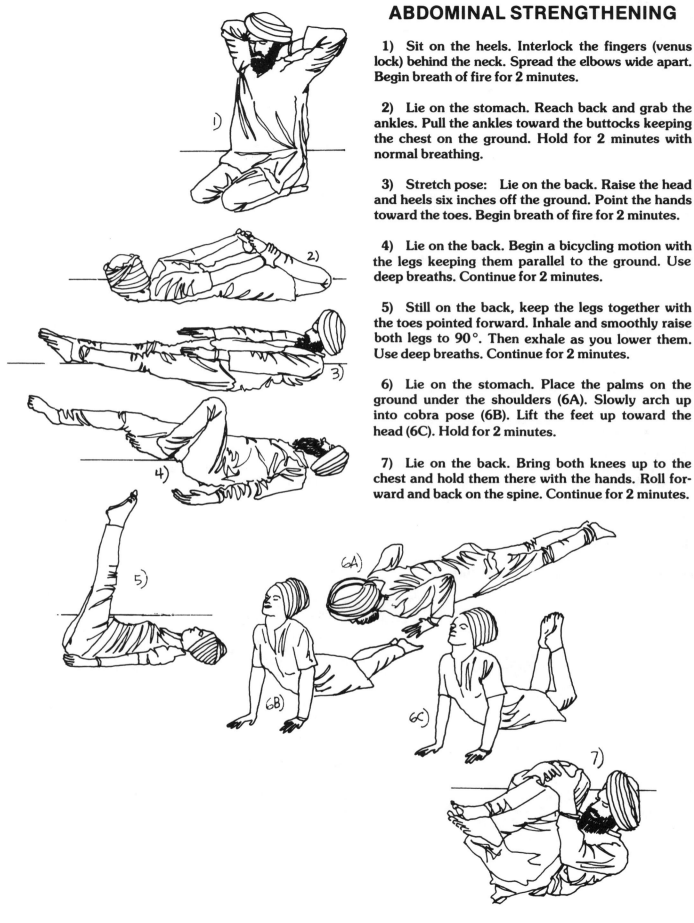

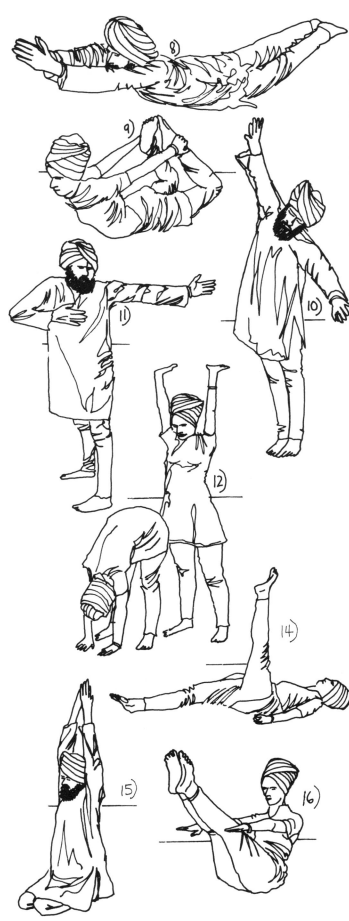

8) Lie on the stomach. Extend the arms forward with the palms flat together. Arch the back so the arms, chest and legs lift off the ground. Hold this extended locust with breath of fire for 2 minutes.

9) Still on the stomach, reach back and grasp the ankles. Arch up into bow pose. Do breath of fire for 2 minutes, then relax.

10) Stand up straight. Keep the legs together. Extend the arms to the sides, parallel to the ground with palms facing down. Without twisting the torso, bend to the left with a deep inhale, then bend to the right with the exhale. Continue this pendulum-like motion for 2 minutes.

11) Still standing, spread the legs 1½ to 2 feet apart. Then swing one arm out to the side, parallel to the ground as the other arm bends in with the palm on the chest. Then switch arms. Inhale as the left arm swings out, exhale as the right arm swings out. Continue for 2 minutes.

12) Still standing, raise both arms straight up with palms facing up (12A). Exhale as you bend forward and try to put the palms on the ground (12B). Inhale as you raise up. Continue for 2 minutes.

13) Lie on the back. Repeat the fourth exercise, the parallel bicycle, for 2 minutes.

14) On the back, inhale while raising the left leg to 90°. Exhale as you lower it. Repeat with the right leg. For 2 minutes, continue this alternate leg lifting with deep breaths.

15) Sit on the heels with the arms stretched up and the palms together. Begin Sat Kriya. Pull in the navel point and say, *"Sat,"* relax the navel point and say *"Nam."* Continue rhythmically for 2 minutes. Then inhale deeply, hold, apply mul bhand. Relax.

16) Sit straight with both legs extended. Lift the legs up 60° from the ground. Extend the arms parallel to the ground with palms down. Begin breath of fire. Continue for 2 minutes. Then totally relax.

COMMENTS:

This kriya gives you a good physical workout. It strengthens the navel point, abdominal muscles, and lower back. It improves circulation. It strengthens the nervous system so that your behavior can be constant and direct. It is an excellent set for strengthening the digestive system.

STRENGTHENING THE AURA

1) **Stand up. Bend forward so the palms are on the ground and the body forms a triangle. Raise the right leg up with the knee straight. Exhale — bend the arms and bring the head near the ground. Inhale — raise up to the original triangle pose. Continue this triangle push-up for 1½ minutes. Switch legs and continue for another 1½ minutes.**

2) Sit in easy pose. Extend the left hand forward as if grasping a pole so the palm faces to the right. Put the right palm facing down crossed under the left wrist (2A). Raise the right hand up over the back of the left hand so both palms face right and the fingers lock (2B). Inhale—raise the arms to 60° (2C). Exhale—bring the arms down to chest level. Keep the elbows straight. Breathe deeply for 2 to 3 minutes. Then inhale—stretch the arms up (2D). Relax.

3) **Put both arms forward, parallel to the ground with palms facing each other about 6 inches apart. As you inhale, let the arms drop back and stretch toward each other. Exhale — bring them forward to the original position. Continue 3 minutes with deep rhythmic breaths.**

COMMENTS:

This is a great kriya for keeping disease away and developing your aura. The time can be built up to 7½ minutes for each side in Exercise 1, and 15 minutes each for Exercises 2 and 3. That will create a tremendous sweat. It will rid almost any digestive problem. It gives strength to the arms and it extends the power of protection and projection in the personality.

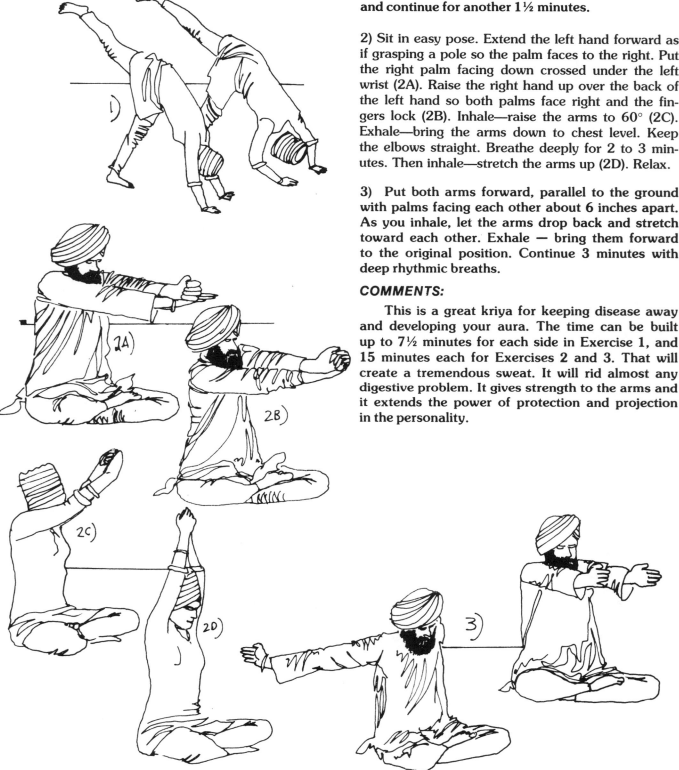

STRENGTH TO SACRIFICE

1) Sit in easy pose with the spine straight and the chest lifted. Put the fingertips together to form a tent-like shape (1A). Hold the hands palms down at the level of the chin (1B). Chant **"God and me, me and God are one."** Keep the fingers pressed tightly together as you chant. Continue for 3 to 6 minutes.

2) Lock the middle fingers of both hands together at chest level. Pull the fingers as hard as you can. Be constant. Hold for 1½ minutes.

3) In easy pose with a straight spine, grasp both wrists with opposite hands (3A). Place this lock behind the neck and pull the hands and forearms down (3B). Hold the position with long deep breathing for 3 minutes.

4) Now grasp the fingertips of each hand by bending the left arm behind the back with palm out, and bending the right arm over the right shoulder. Then inhale, exhale deeply, hold the breath out and pull the navel lock tightly. For 3 minutes, repeat the breath and lock cycle.

5) Stretch the legs out straight. Bend forward and grab the toes. Hold as still as a rock for 10 seconds. Then relax.

COMMENTS:

The capacity to transcend the sacrifice of the body is required of the yogi and the saint. For this the nerves must be strong and balanced. The circumvent magnetic force of the aura must be so strong that no negativity can enter your field. The ability to teach well requires the capacity to speak directly only to receptive ears. You need the strength not to be provoked to answers by foolish discussion. Your words should be pure. A sense of reality sometimes comes in the transcendence of minor pains. This kriya helps conquer two great negative gifts of man: the ability and tendency to escape from situations, self commitment, and the abliity to hear only what we want to hear.

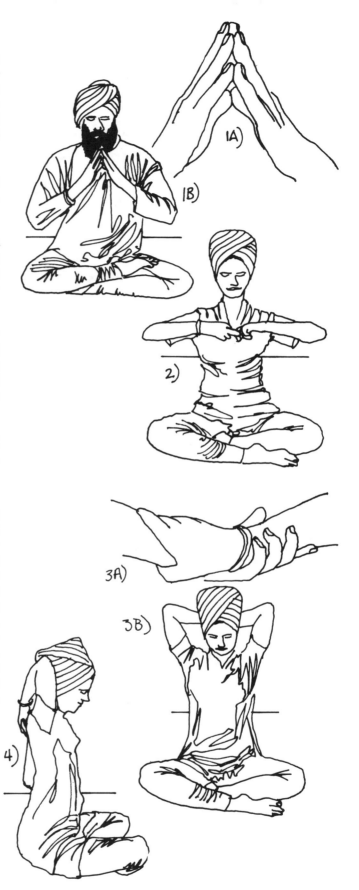

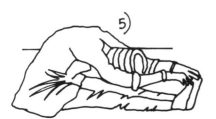

KRIYA FOR NERVE, NAVEL, AND LOWER SPINE STRENGTH

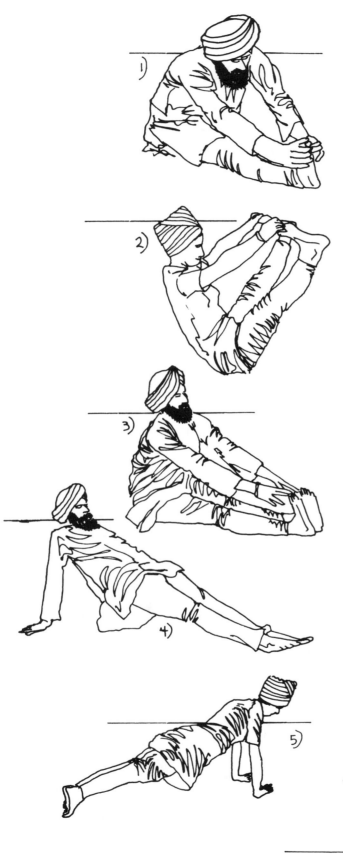

1)   Sit with the left heel at the rectum and the right leg extended straight forward. Bend forward and grasp the toes with both hands. Straighten the spine and look forward to the toes. Stay perfectly still with normal breathing. Keep a light mul bhand applied. Continue for 3 minutes. Then inhale deeply and pull back on the toes. Completely exhale, pull back more and apply a strong mul bhand. Repeat this deep breath 2 more times. Relax.

2)   Come into the kundalini lotus pose: Balance on the sacrum by holding the toes of both feet, spreading the legs wide, and raising the legs off the ground 60°. Keep the spine straight. Apply a constant mul bhand. Use normal breathing. Hold for 3 minutes. Then inhale deeply, exhale and apply a strong mul bhand. Repeat the deep breath 2 more times. Relax.

3)   Extend both legs straight. Reach forward and hold onto the toes. Pull the spine up straight by pulling back on the toes. Pull the chin straight back. Begin long deep breaths. Continue for 3 minutes. Then apply a strong mul bhand on the exhale of a deep breath. Repeat mul bhand 2 more times.

4)   Form a back platform pose: keep the legs extended straight. Put the palms on the ground behind you. Lift the stomach and buttocks up until the body is straight with only the heels and palms on the ground. Bring the chin to the chest. Press the toes forward. Hold the position with normal breathing. Continue for 3 minutes. Inhale deeply, exhale and apply mul bhand. Repeat the breath 2 more times. Relax.

5)   Lie on the stomach. Put the palms on the ground under the shoulders. Push up off the ground with the body straight until you form a front platform. Exhale as you slowly go down to the ground. Inhale as you slowly rise up. Do not apply mul bhand. Continue with deep, slow breaths 26 times. Relax.

6)   Lie on the back. Raise up on the elbows. Place the elbows under the shoulders. Raise the buttocks up so the spine and body are straight. Only the heels

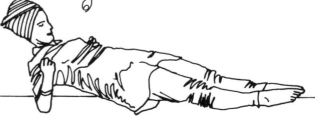

and elbows are on the ground. Press the toes forward. Hold the pose with long deep breathing. Continue for 3 minutes. Then exhale completely and apply mul bhand.

7) Sit on the heels. Slowly lean back until the head and possibly the shoulders are on the ground. The arms are relaxed on the ground beside the legs. Keep a light, constant mul bhand applied. Begin deep breaths. Continue for 3 minutes. Then exhale completely, and apply a strong mul bhand. Inhale. Repeat the complete exhale and mul bhand 2 more times. Relax.

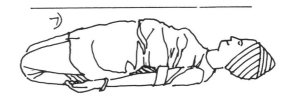

8) Come into frog pose: squat down with the toes on the ground, the heels together off the ground, and the fingers on the ground between spread knees. Inhale — raise the buttocks up as the head goes down. Exhale — squat down to the original position Continue with deep breaths 30 times.

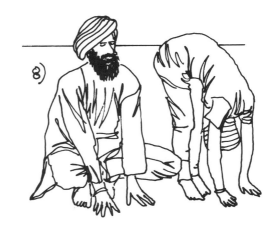

9) Lie on the back. Place the arms relaxed along the sides with the palms up. Inhale — lift one leg up to 90°. Exhale — let it down smoothly to the ground. Switch legs with each breath cycle. With each inhale apply a slight mul bhand. Continue for 3 minutes.

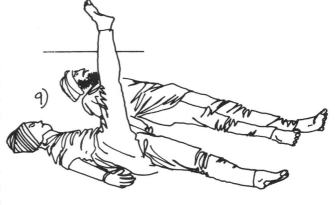

10) Sit in a comfortable meditation posture. Pull in the navel point and apply mul bhand. Mentally view the entire body. Then negate each identity that comes to mind: "I am not a man, not a woman, not a student, not a teacher, not sitting, etc." You are not the body, mind, or spirit but the consciousness that gives rise to and integrates them all. Continue at least 3 minutes.

COMMENTS:

This kriya is not recommended for early beginners. It is a good physical workout that requires flexibility and endurance. The lower nerve plexi are pressured and the vital energy is raised above the diaphragm. This set is of great value for any consistent difficulty with digestion or elimination. If you get very nervous and shaky under tense situations, this set is excellent. It is an excellent preparatory kriya for meditations that release you from false identifications to the body or mind.

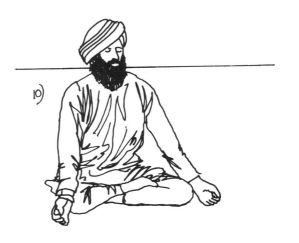

STRENGTHENING THE INNER LIGHT

1) Sit in easy pose with a straight spine. Place the hands in gyan mudra with straight arms resting on the knees. Close the eyelids and focus deeply. Inhale and exhale deeply. This cycle will take about 8 seconds. Take a total of 12 breaths. On the thirteenth breath cycle, exhale completely and hold the breath out. Pump the stomach in and out at a moderate pace. (You may add a mentally repeated *"Sat"* as you pull the belly in, and *"Nam"* as you relax it and push it out.) When you can no longer hold the breath out, repeat the exercise. Continue for 3 minutes.

2) Stretch the legs forward. Keep the spine erect. Bend the right leg so the right foot rests on top of the left thigh at the hip-groin level. Bend forward at the waist and grasp the toes of the left foot with both hands. Keep the spine as straight as you can and look toward the toes. Breathe long and deeply. As you breathe, constrict the tip of your nose as if you were "sniffing." Continue for 3 minutes. Then inhale, hold briefly, and relax.

3) Sit straight and meditate on the calm flow of the breath. Briefly visualize your spine from the base to the top and then to the brow point. Relax and meditate.

COMMENTS:

This kriya helps you gain endurance and constancy. The first exercise stimulates the navel center and digestion. The second exercise gives energy to the upper body and stretches the life nerves in the legs. The third allows the energy changes to stabilize and consolidate themselves.

In life, we must increase our wisdom and experience so we can live normally but with higher consciousness. The yogic aim is to live with maximum light and effectiveness but also very humbly. This is why a teacher remains a student throughout his life and grows more humble with age. This kriya lets the Self take care of the gross self so that the physical body can have the energy to carry out the Self's desires. Regular practice of this kriya helps balance the difference between your inner reality and your expression. A good way to practice this kriya is to repeat the set 3 to 4 times, then deeply relax for 5 to 10 minutes.

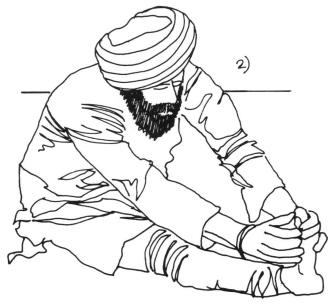

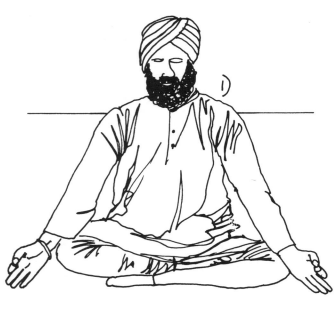

KRIYA FOR TOLERANCE

1) Sit in easy pose with the spine straight. Lock the fingertips together like hooks with the right palm facing down. Push the side of the hands into the belly. As you press the hands in, exhale completely, hold the breath out, then inhale and hold the breath for 7 to 8 seconds. Continue this cycle for 3 minutes.

2) Sit on the heels and raise the arms over the head with palms flat together. Pull in the navel point as you say **"Sat,"** relax the navel point as you say **"Nam."** Continue Sat Kriya for 3 minutes.

3) Stretch the legs out straight in front of you. Place the palms on the ground in back of the hips. Raise both legs to a 60° angle from the ground. Hold this position and begin breath of fire. Continue for 2 minutes, then inhale, exhale, apply mul bhand. Relax immediately into easy pose and belly laugh loudly for 1 minute.

4) Sit in easy pose. Hold both arms bent with the hands as fists at shoulder height. Inhale deeply and hold the breath. As you hold, begin punching forward (as in boxing) with alternate hands. When you must, exhale and inhale deeply. Continue for 3 minutes.

5) Sit in easy pose. Alternate between camel ride and shoulder lifts; put the hands on the shins. In-hale — press the spine forward (5A). Exhale — push it back (5B). Inhale — lift the shoulders up to the ears (5C). Exhale — let the shoulders down (5D). Continue this cycle with deep breaths for 3 minutes. Then inhale, exhale completely, apply mul bhand. Relax.

COMMENTS:

To gain strength for tolerance and humility, the navel center needs to be developed. This kriya works on the abdomen, stimulating the navel energy to rise to the higher centers and then integrating it with the whole aura. It is a good preparation for meditation. Two cycles of this kriya give you a physical tune-up.

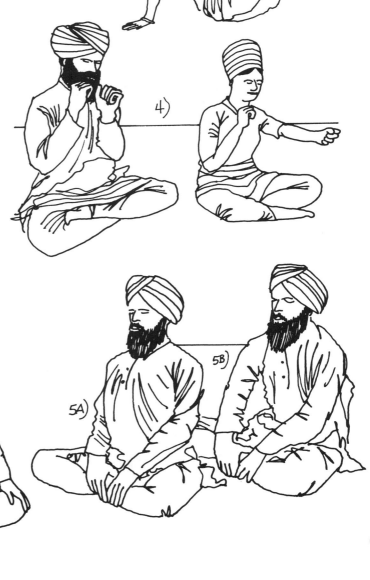

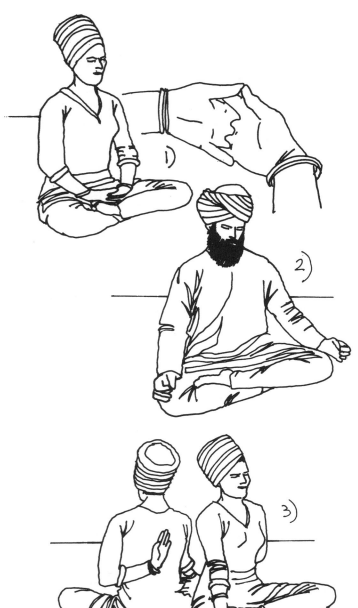

DISEASE RESISTANCE AND HEART HELPER

1) Sit in easy pose. Interlace the fingers of both hands. Press the thumb tips together. Put this hand lock with palms up in the lap. Apply mul bhand by contracting and pulling up the rectum, pulling in the navel point, and lifting up the sex organ. Chant *"God and me, me and God are one."* With each cycle of the mantra, pull up the locks a little tighter. Continue for 3 minutes.

2) Sit in easy pose with the hands in gyan mudra resting on the knees. Inhale deeply, exhale slowly and completely without dropping the rib cage. Hold the breath out and pump the stomach in and out. When you cannot pump anymore, take another breath and continue for 3 minutes.

3) Sit in easy pose. Bring the left arm in back of the torso. Bend at the elbow and stretch the left hand toward the right shoulder. The palm faces away from the body. Inhale deeply, exhale completely. Hold the breath out as long as you can. Apply mul bhand. Then inhale and repeat the cycle. Continue 3 to 5 minutes.

4) Sit in any comfortable meditation posture. Meditate on the regular energetic flow of the breath. Feel your radiance and light.

COMMENTS:

The first exercise improves your health by invigorating the first chakra and elimination. It promotes calmness and disease resistance. The third chakra, endurance, and nerve strength are stimulated by Exercise 2. Exercise 3 strengthens the heart and increases circulation above the diaphragm. Three repetitions of this kriya is a very effective practice.

CIRCULATORY SYSTEMS AND MAGNETIC FIELD

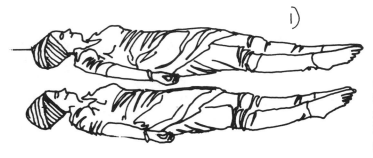

1) Lie down flat on the back, arms straight along the thighs, heels and toes together. Press the toes forward. Press the toes deeper and deeper for 1 minute, then lift the heels 6 inches. Begin long deep breathing. Keep the head relaxed down on the ground and continue for 3 minutes.

2) Dead relaxation for 2 minutes.

3) Again press the toes forward with the hands straight along the thighs and toes pressed down maximumly. Hold for 1 minute. Now lift the heels up 3 inches only. Apply mul bhand. Relax.

4) Dead relaxation. Become disassociated from the body. Imagine that there are no legs, no arms, no trunk, no head. Continue for 2 minutes.

5) Sit in easy pose. Put hands on shoulders in a "U" with fingers in front, thumbs in back. Begin breathing long and deep for 3 minutes, then inhale and mentally circulate the pranic energy. Relax.

6) Make an antenna of the right hand with fingers straight up in the air and the thumb closing off the right nostril. Begin long deep breathing through the left nostril for 5 minutes. Inhale — hold for 30 seconds and let the energy circulate in the body. Exhale.

7) Lie on the back. Lift toes and head 12 inches from the ground. KEEP UP! Do normal breathing for 2 minutes and breath of fire for 1 more minute to relieve pain. Inhale — hold, and relax.

8) Deep relaxation to a gong or to the chanting of long "*Sat Nam's*" (see "Basic Breath Series"), or any beautiful divine version of the *Ashtang Mantra* can be done. Relax for 10 minutes. Then rotate the wrists and ankles and stretch the spine.

9) Lie with hands at sides and legs straight together. Begin bundle roll. Imagine the body is a bundle of logs tied together and roll over and over without using the arms or legs, like logs rolling downhill.

10) Without a rest, lie flat on the back, open the mouth, and laugh loudly. Release the energy through the lungs. Relax for 1 minute and laugh again. Relax.

COMMENTS:

Blood is the life supply line to your cells. Did you know that the blood cells act differently with different magnetic influences? Exercises 1-4 raise and lower the blood pressure and increase circulation to the limbs and head. Exercises 5-7 magnetize and charge the blood with pranic force. This is like getting a transfusion of fresh young blood. The last exercise allows the new energy to circulate and affect the entire body. With the bundle roll, you consolidate those effects for the rest of the day.

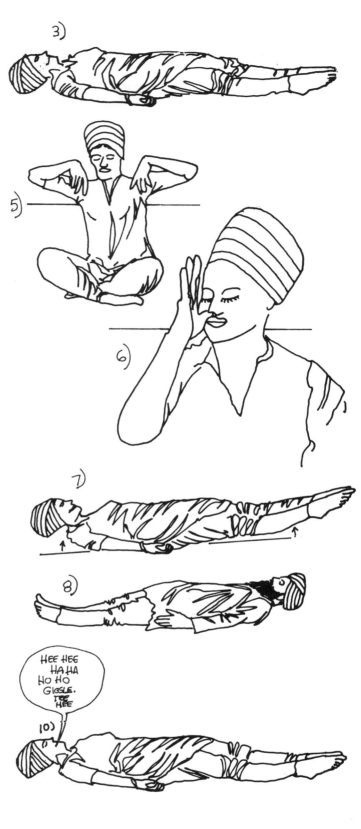

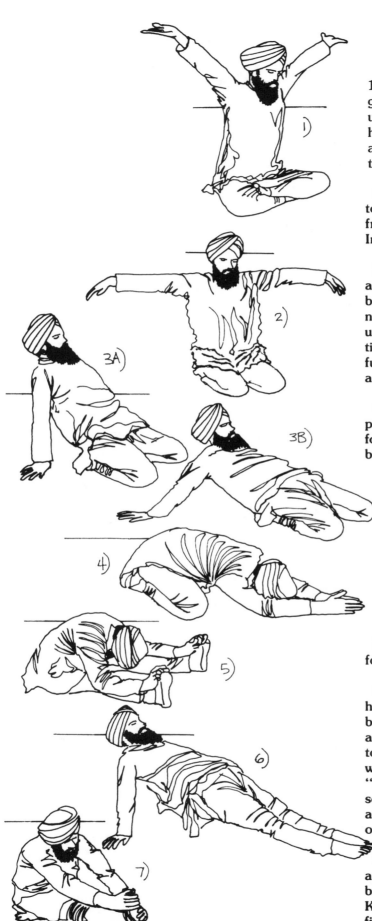

MAGNETIC FIELD AND HEART CENTER

1) Sit in easy pose. Hold the arms up at a 60° angle with wrists and elbows straight, palms facing up (1A). Begin breath of fire for 1 minute. Then inhale—hold the breath and pump the stomach in and out 16 times. Exhale—relax the breath. Continue the cycle for 2 to 3 minutes.

2) Immediately sit on the heels with arms parallel to the ground at the sides. Let the hands hang limp from the wrists. Begin breath of fire for 3 minutes. Inhale — hold, and relax.

3) Sit on the heels. Spread the knees wide apart and lean back 60° from the ground. Support the body with arms straight down in back (3A). Tilt the neck back — inhale — pump the stomach in and out until the breath can be held no longer. Exhale. Continue for 1½ to 2 minutes. Then, tilt the spine back further to 30° and continue the breathing cycle for another 1½ to 2 minutes (3B).

4) Still sitting on the heels with knees widespread, put the forehead on the ground with arms stretched forward and relaxed. After 1 minute, begin long deep breathing for 2 minutes. Then for 2 minutes chant:

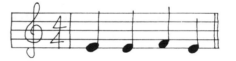

*Teacher: "**Ong, ong, ong, ong.**"*
*Class: "**Ong, ong, ong, ong.**"*
*Teacher: "**Sohung, sohung, sohung, sohung.**"*
*Class: "**Sohung, sohung, sohung, sohung.**"*

5) Grab the toes with legs slightly spread. Hold for 1 minute.

6) Back platform: The body is straight with the heels on the ground and the upper portion of the body held up by straight arms. Drop the head back and begin breath of fire. After 30 seconds, begin to "walk" the legs wider apart until they are spread wide. Walk them back together again and continue "walking" while doing breath of fire for 30 more seconds. Inhale, exhale and move immediately into a front stretch holding the toes for 1 minute. Relax on back for 3 minutes.

7) Sit on the left heel, stretch the right leg forward and grab the big toe with the right hand. Pulling back on the toe, grab the heel with the left hand. Keep the chin tucked into the chest and the eyes fixed on the big toe. Inhale deeply — exhale and

hold the breath out for 8 seconds keeping mul bhand and diaphragm lock tightly pulled. Inhale. Continue for 3 minutes. Relax for 5 minutes on the back.

8) Lie on the back. Stretch the arms overhead on the ground. Raise the left leg 90° and begin breath of fire for 1 minute (8A). Switch to the right leg for 1 minute, continuing breath of fire. Then raise both legs 12 inches only and keep up the breath of fire for 1 more minute (8B). Relax for 2 minutes.

9) Slowly come into shoulder stand. Spread the legs wide open and begin breath of fire for 3 minutes. Relax on the back for 3 minutes.

10) Lie on the back. Inhale and lift both legs six inches. Arms should be straight up from the shoulders with the palms facing in (10A). On the exhale, let both legs down and bring the head up pressing the chin on the chest (10B). Continue 3 minutes with long deep breathing. Relax 2 minutes.

11) Sit in easy pose and hold opposite elbows across the chest. Roll the head in a slow figure 8 for 30 seconds in one direction, then 30 seconds in the other direction. Then inhale deeply, and bend forward to the ground. Exhale and rise up as fast as possible. Repeat this 10 times.

12) Meditate by chanting:

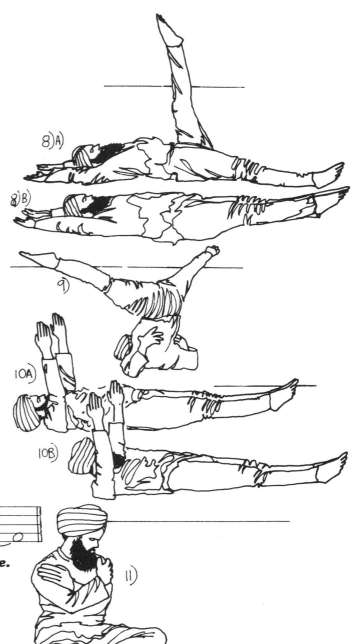

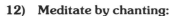
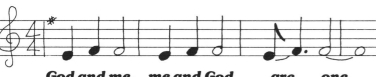

God and me, me and God, are one.

COMMENTS:

This set works on coordination and repair of the nervous system by stimulating the heart center. Your normal feeling of happiness, connection, and well-being depend on the balance of your individual psycho-electromagnetic field. If it is strong, your muscles obey the message nerves, and the message nerves give good perception to the brain. Proper maintenance of the nerves depends on the basic elements and hormones in the constitution of the blood. This set will balance the blood.

Exercise 1 builds the psycho-electromagnetic field. If your elbows bend, the psycho-electromagnetic field will not be reformed and strengthened properly. If the exhale after pumping the stomach is rough or gasping, then your magnetic field is very weak. The second exercise is for the heart. This stimulates the thyroid, parathyroid and navel center. If you practice these, you will never need cosmetics. A smooth, radiant complexion and a glow in the eyes and face is a natural by-product of this exercise.

Exercise 4 feeds the newly-constituted blood into the brain cells and moves the spinal fluid. This helps repair the damage to the brain done by drugs like alcohol, marijuana, etc. Exercise 5 is for balance and 6 is for the thyroid, lower back and heart. Exercise 7 is the great seal of yoga: Maha mudra. Its effects fill pages. This exercise can be practiced by itself. Exercise 8 balances prana and apana. Exercise 9 is for the thyroid and 10 and 11 are for the heart center.

The best results are always obtained if you practice a set until you master it. If you cannot do the exercises for the full time period, do what you can and slowly build up to it. When you can keep up on all the given times and are in a good posture for each exercise, continue the set each day for 40 days as you master the mental poise and meditation of the full set.

VARUYAS KRIYA

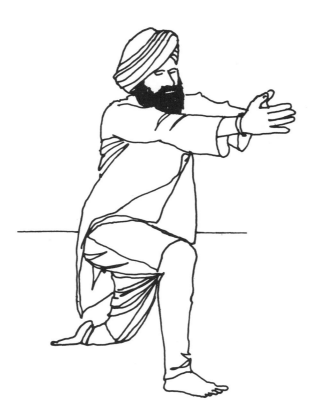

Stand up straight. Put the right foot slightly forward. Stretch the left leg far backward. Put the top of the toes of the left foot on the ground. Extend the arms forward parallel to the ground. Put the palms together. Tilt the spine slightly forward of the vertical position. Fix the eyes on the horizon or at the brow point.

Take a deep breath, then begin a rhythmic chant of *"Sat Nam."* Emphasize the sound *"Sat"* as you pull the navel point in and apply a light mul bhand. Continue for 1½ minutes. Then inhale. Relax.

Switch and place the left leg forward. Repeat the exercise for an equal period of time.

COMMENTS:

This kriya will make you sweat if you do it properly. You may also notice a burning sensation in the cheeks. The time of practice can slowly be increased to 7½ minutes on each side. The practice and perfection of this kriya is said to open the pituitary secretion, regulate excessive sexual energy, and increase general immunity to disease. It tests the nerve strength and rebalances the magnetic field of the body. If you don't want to be shaky when you are older, this is an excellent practice to start when you are young. Besides practicing this kriya by itself, it is enjoyable to do it after completing a long series of exercises that have worked on flexibility and circulation. The kriya helps transform the "vital juice," the *ojas*, into a form usable in maintaining your entire nervous system.

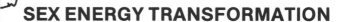

SEX ENERGY TRANSFORMATION

1) Lie on the stomach. Place the hands on the ground directly under the shoulders (1A). Arch the neck back and lift up into cobra pose (1B). Inhale and raise the hips straight off the ground coming into a front platform pose (1C). Exhale as the hips go back down into cobra pose. Repeat 26 times, then relax 2 minutes on the stomach. The teacher should chant *"Ong"* — the infinite, creative consciousness, on the inhale; and *"Sohung"* — I am Thou, on the exhale. This will keep a rhythm and keep the mind focused.

2) Come into cow pose (2A). Stretch forward with an exhale making the hips and chin touch the ground. Keep the head up and arms bent (2B). Inhale back into cow pose. The teacher chants *"Ong-Sohung"*: *"Ong"* on the forward motion, *"Sohung"* on resuming cow pose. Repeat 26 times.

3) Immediately without resting, lie on the back. Bend the knees and hold the ankles with the hands. The soles of the feet should stay on the ground next to the buttocks (3A). Inhale — raise the hips up (3B). Exhale — bring them down. Repeat 26 times, rest for 2 minutes, and repeat 26 more times.

4) Immediately lie down on the back. Raise both legs 18 inches and start long deep powerful breathing for 30 seconds. Bring one knee to the chest, then the other with each deep inhale. Continue alternating with this push-pull action for 45 seconds to 1 minute. Inhale — hold both legs straight out for 5 seconds. Relax.

5) Lie on the back. Bring the soles of the feet together and grab them with the hands. Rock back and forth for 30-45 seconds.

6) Deep relaxation for 2 minutes.

7) Stretch pose: Hold the feet and head 6 inches off the ground with normal breathing. The eyes are fixed on the toes. Balance in this position and hold it for up to 7 minutes. Inhale deeply, exhale, hold the breath out and apply mul bandh. Hold the breath out as long as possible. Repeat the inhale, exhale, hold, and mul bandh 4 more times. Then relax down.

8) Completely relax for 5 minutes letting the energy circulate. Think of God and God consciousness. Feel unlimited. Then, lying on your back, repeat out loud: *"God and me, me and God, are one"* about 12 times, raising the pitch and volume frequently. Inhale deeply, hold for 15 seconds, then exhale. Start the chant again but *very powerfully*. Chant loudly from the solar plexus. The eyes should be closed. Do not feel shy. Inhale and exhale deeply eight times, then inhale holding the breath in and raise both legs 90° for 15 seconds. Exhale and relax.

9) Sit in Sidhasana (perfect pose), or Sukasan (easy pose). Use the tip of the thumb and the tip of the little finger of one hand to close alternate nostrils. Inhale through the left nostril, exhale through the right. Meditate at the base of the spine and pull mul bandh. On the inhale, think "**Sat**," the Truth; on the exhale vibrate "**Nam**," the Identity or Name. Continue for 1 minute. Then begin breath of fire in through the left nostril, out through the right for 1 minute. Without a break, inhale and exhale through the left nostril only, moderately fast for about 15 seconds. Begin breath of fire through the left nostril for 15 seconds, then through the right nostril for 15 seconds, then breathe again 5 seconds through the left and 5 seconds through the right nostril. Inhale through both nostrils and hold 5 seconds. Exhale, holding the breath out and mentally repeat "**Sat Nam**," making the sound follow an upward spiral up

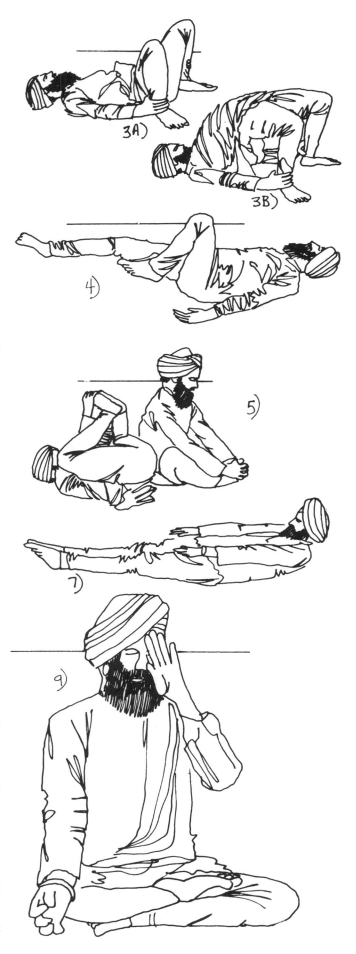

3A)

3B)

4)

5)

7)

9)

the spine for 30 seconds. Then visualize the "**Sat**" going down both sides of the spine, entering the base of the spine, and "**Nam**" rising up the middle of the spine. Hold the mind against every other thing and concentrate. NOW is the time. Inhale deeply. Exhale. Repeat the mental meditation one more time.

10) Chant "*Ek Ong Kar Sat Nam Sat Nam Siri Wahe Guru*" in the following manner:

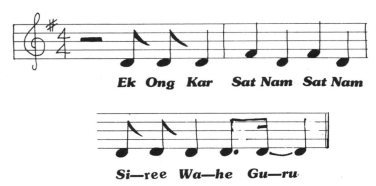

Ek Ong Kar   Sat Nam Sat Nam

Si—ree Wa—he Gu—ru

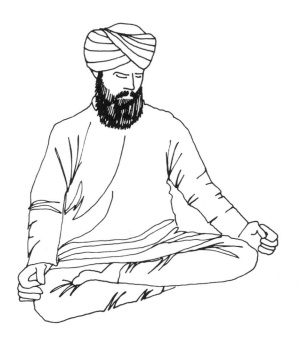

When chanting "**Sat Nam**" and "**Guru**" apply and release mul bandh. Gradually the mul bandh will become so strong and locked that it will be easy to hold throughout the entire chant. Continue chanting for 6 minutes. Inhale—hold for 15 seconds. Relax or meditate.

COMMENTS:

In our culture, we are taught to view sex in terms of pleasure and reproduction. We are not educated in the need for moderation in sex in order to maintain our health and nerve balance. Sexual experience in the correct consciousness can give you the experience of God and bliss, but before that can ever occur you must charge your sexual batteries and possess a real potency. The seminal fluids produced in the male and female contain high concentrations of minerals and elements that are crucial to proper nerve balance and brain functioning. The sexual fluid is reabsorbed by the body if it is allowed to mature. Its essence, or *ojas,* is transported into the spinal fluid. Running your mind without the ojas is like running a car without oil — you wear out quickly. About 90% of your sexual energy is used to repair and rejuvenate the organs of the body. The normal span of potency for a yogi is equal to the length of his life. In the United States, potency wanes even in the early forties. This kriya will generate sexual energy and transmute it into ojas and healing force.

The first three exercises activate the sex chakra; then the navel point and lower spine. Exercise 3 is especially effective for relieving tension and problems of the ovaries. Exercise 4 and 5 move the energy out of the digestive system. Exercise 7 distributes the energy from the navel point above the solar plexus to the heart center. Exercise 9 uses pranayam to completely open your psychic channels and move the kundalini energy all the way to the highest chakras. Exercise 10 uses the Kundalini energy in the mantra to project the mind into the infinity of the cosmos and beyond the normal earthly consciousness.

BREATH MEDITATION SERIES FOR GLANDULAR BALANCE

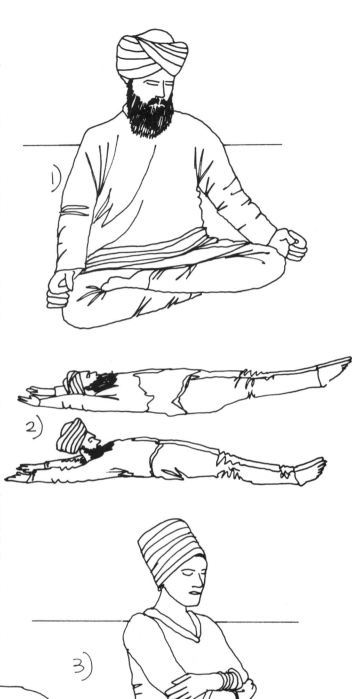

1) Sit in easy pose. Break your inhale into 16 short sniffs. With each sniff, mentally vibrate *"Sat Nam."* When you exhale break the breath 16 times, again mentally vibrating *"Sat Nam."* With this continuous breathing pull the navel point slightly with each sniff. Start with 5 minutes of practice. Then add 1 minute each day to a maximum of 31 minutes.

2) Lie on the back. Put the arms straight overhead on the ground with the palms up. Inhale — raise both legs 6 inches. Exhale — let the legs down and press the chin to the chest. Continue with long deep breathing for 3 minutes. Then rest for 2 minutes.

3) Sit in easy pose. Grab your elbows with the arms across the chest. Inhale — raise to a straight sitting position. Exhale — bend forward and put the forehead to the ground. Continue for 3 minutes with long deep breaths.

COMMENTS:

Your glands are the guardians of your physical health and your stability in infinite consciousness. Their secretions determine the chemistry of the blood and the blood, in turn, determines the composition of your personality. If, for example, you lack proper iodine from the thyroid gland, you will lack patience and seldom succeed in staying calm and cool.

If you are to gain mastery of unlimited consciousness in yourself you must master the physical consciousness to help you, not hinder you. It is best to work on this while you are young. Once you are old, it is too late to take care of old age. Prepare your glandular balance now so that age, disease, and fatigue may not blunt the enjoyment of the God-consciousness you are building.

If you keep the first exercise to 5 minutes, then just repeat the kriya 3 times to have a thorough glandular workout.

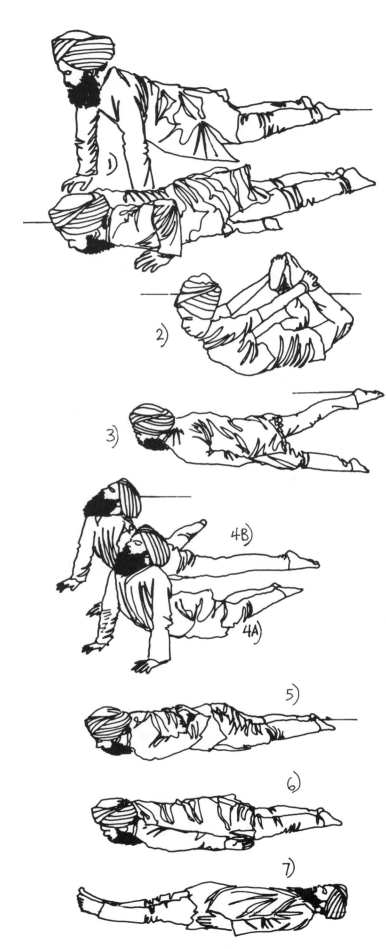

RESERVE ENERGY SET

1) Lie on the stomach, heels together. Inhale—rise up to a push-up position. Only the upper side of the bent toes and the palms remain on the ground. Exhale down. Continue 15 times up and down in a moderately slow rhythm.

2) Lie on the stomach. Reach back and grab the ankles, stretching up into bow pose. Begin breath of fire for 30 seconds. Inhale, exhale, and relax on the stomach, hands straight at the sides.

3) Lie on stomach. Make fists of the hands and place them below the waistline just above and inside the bend of the legs. Inhale — raise the left leg up. Exhale — raise the right as the left is lowered. Continue alternating with the breath for 2 minutes.

4) Relax into cobra pose. Hold the pose, but just relax (4A). Heels are together, arms straight, head back. Relax in this posture 45 seconds, then spread the legs far apart and bring the hands closer into the body to create a deeper back bend (4B). Roll the head back and forth by turning the chin from the right shoulder to the left shoulder, inhaling at the right and exhaling at the left. Continue 4 or 5 times.

5) Relax and lie down on the stomach, grabbing the wrists behind the back. Roll left and right on the chest with the legs straight and heels together. Continue for 30 seconds.

6) In the same position with arms straight along the sides, begin relaxing each part of the body. Go deep within yourself for 5 minutes.

7) Bundle roll: Lie straight on the back with arms at the sides like a bundle of logs tied together. Flip yourself over and over from back to stomach, stomach to back without bending the body, arms or legs. *Do not bend anywhere.* Continue for 3 minutes.

8) Total relaxation on back for 10 minutes.

COMMENTS:

To tap the reserve flow of the kundalini energy in your body, you activate the sexual energy in exercise 1, the navel energy in 2 and 3, and move that energy up the spine in 4A. During exercise 4B, the thyroid gland secretes and opens circulation to the upper brain. This clears your thinking and adds energy to the will. The last two exercises charge and strengthen your electromagnetic field and stabilize the new energy state you have created. This set gives you an extra resistance to the fluctuations of the environment.

PURIFYING THE SELF

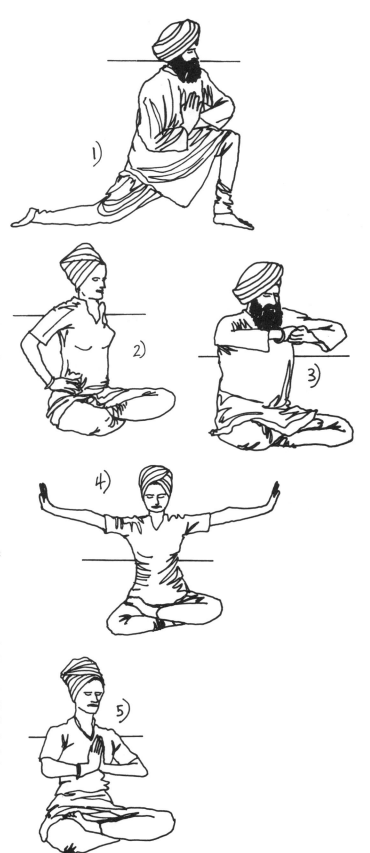

1) Stand up. Then squat down, keeping the feet flat. Extend one leg back as far as you can with the top of the foot on the ground. Most of the pressure will be on the bent leg. Put the palms together at the level of the mind nerve at the center of the chest. Focus on the brow point. Inhale deeply and hold for 7 to 8 seconds. Repeat this cycle 3 times. Then switch legs and do it completely again. Continue until each leg has been extended back 3 times.

2) Sit in easy pose. Lift the diaphragm high. Raise both shoulders as high as possible. Place the hands on the hips. Inhale and exhale very deeply while holding this posture. Continue 2 to 3 minutes.

3) Still in easy pose, hook the fingers together at the center of the chest with the right palm facing down. Forearms and elbows are parallel to the ground. Inhale deeply. Exhale completely with force and apply mul bhand. Inhale — hold the breath, apply mul bhand and mentally raise the pranic energy from the base of the spine to the top. Continue this breath cycle for 3 minutes.

4) Sit in easy pose. Extend the arms out from the sides, parallel to the ground. Press the fingers up, palms facing out. Roll the eyes up and focus at the brow point. Inhale deeply — hold the breath while applying a firm mul bhand for 20 seconds. Then exhale and repeat the cycle. Continue for 2 to 3 minutes.

5) In easy pose, press the palms together with the fingers pointing up. Pull the spine straight. Press the palms together with 30 to 50 pounds of pressure. Hold the position for 2 minutes. Then relax.

COMMENTS:

This kriya energizes you and helps purify the mind and body. It is an excellent kriya to practice before giving a healing-relaxing massage to someone. If you massage people professionally, it can keep your energy together and prevent you from getting drained. Exercise 1 will raise the sexual and digestive energies of the body. Exercise 2 will open the lungs and thyroid. Exercise 3 opens the heart and gives it strength. Exercises 4 and 5 increase healing power in the hands and circulation to the upper body.

SURYA KRIYA

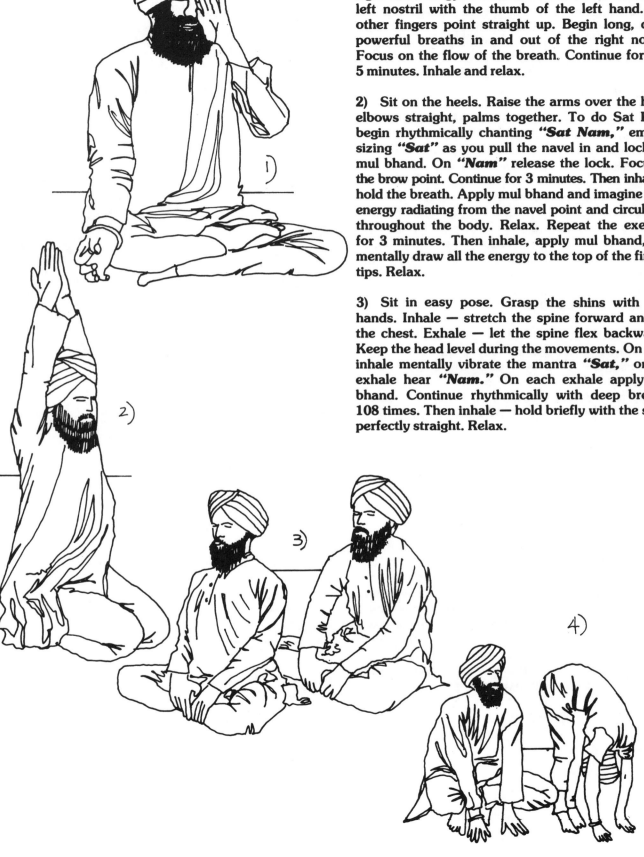

1) Sit in easy pose with a straight spine. Rest the right hand in gyan mudra on the knee. Block the left nostril with the thumb of the left hand. The other fingers point straight up. Begin long, deep, powerful breaths in and out of the right nostril. Focus on the flow of the breath. Continue for 3 to 5 minutes. Inhale and relax.

2) Sit on the heels. Raise the arms over the head, elbows straight, palms together. To do Sat Kriya begin rhythmically chanting *"Sat Nam,"* emphasizing *"Sat"* as you pull the navel in and lock the mul bhand. On *"Nam"* release the lock. Focus at the brow point. Continue for 3 minutes. Then inhale — hold the breath. Apply mul bhand and imagine your energy radiating from the navel point and circulating throughout the body. Relax. Repeat the exercise for 3 minutes. Then inhale, apply mul bhand, and mentally draw all the energy to the top of the fingertips. Relax.

3) Sit in easy pose. Grasp the shins with both hands. Inhale — stretch the spine forward and lift the chest. Exhale — let the spine flex backwards. Keep the head level during the movements. On each inhale mentally vibrate the mantra *"Sat,"* on the exhale hear *"Nam."* On each exhale apply mul bhand. Continue rhythmically with deep breaths 108 times. Then inhale — hold briefly with the spine perfectly straight. Relax.

4) Come into frog pose: Place the toes on the ground, the heels together off the ground, the fingers on the ground between the knees, and lift the head up. Inhale — raise the buttocks high. Lower the forehead toward the knees and keep the heels off the ground. Exhale — come back to the original squatting position. Continue with deep breaths 26 times. Inhale up, then relax down onto the heels.

5) Sitting on the heels, place the hands on the thighs. With the spine very straight, inhale deeply and turn the head to the left. Mentally vibrate *"Sat."* Exhale completely as you turn the head to the right. Mentally vibrate *"Nam."* Continue inhaling and exhaling for 3 minutes. Then inhale with the head straight forward. Relax.

6) Sit in easy pose. Put the hands on the shoulders with the fingers in front and the thumbs in the back. The upper arms and elbows are parallel to the ground. Inhale as you bend to the left, exhale and bend to the right. Continue this swaying motion with deep breaths for 3 minutes. Then inhale straight. Relax.

7) Sit in a perfect meditative posture with the spine straight. Direct all attention through the brow point. Pull the navel point in — hold it — apply mul bhand.

Watch the flow of breath. On the inhale listen to silent *"Sat,"* on the exhale listen to silent *"Nam."* Continue 6 minutes or longer.

COMMENTS:

This kriya is named after the energy of the sun. When you have a lot of "sun energy" you do not get cold, you are energetic, expressive, extroverted and enthusiastic. It is the energy of purification. It holds the weight down. It aids digestion. It makes the mind clear, analytic, and action-oriented. The exercises systematically stimulate the positive pranic force and the kundalini energy itself. Exercise 1 draws on the "sun" breath and gives you a clear, focused mind. Exercise 2 is for the release of the energy stored at the navel point. Exercise 3 brings the released kundalini energy along the path of the spine and aids its flexibility. Exercise 4 transforms the sexual energy. Exercise 5 opens the throat chakra, stimulates circulation to the head and works on the thyroid and parathyroid glands. Exercise 6 flexes the spine, distributes the energy over the whole body, and balances the magnetic field. Exercise 7 takes you into a deep self-healing meditation. This should occasionally be in your regular sadhana practice to build the strength of your body and your ability to focus on many tasks.

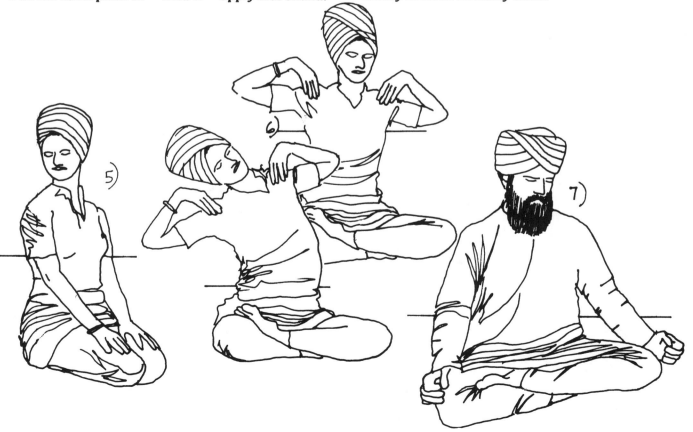

KRIYA FOR CONQUERING SLEEP

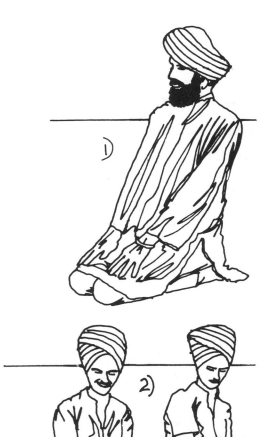

1) Sit on the heels with the palms on the thighs. Keep the spine straight and lean back 30° from the vertical position. Hold the posture with long deep breathing for 1 minute. Then relax.

2) Still sitting on the heels, fold the arms across the chest and hold onto the elbows. Rotate the torso in a circle from right to left. Continue this grinding motion for 3 minutes.

3) Immediately stretch the legs out straight. Put the hands on the ground next to the hips. With the inhale lift the heels and body off the ground. With the exhale drop the body. Do 20 of these "body drops" with the breath.

4) Repeat Exercise 2 for 3 minutes.

5) Repeat Exercise 3 for 15 body drops.

6) Come into bridge pose: Raise the hips up and bend at the knees. The palms and feet are on the ground. Let the head relax back. Hold the pose for 1 minute with normal breathing. Continue with breath of fire for 3 minutes. Inhale, exhale completely, and hold the breath out as you apply mul bhand. Relax.

7) Repeat Exercise 3 for 10 body drops.

8) Repeat Exercise 6 (bridge pose) for 3 minutes with breath of fire.

9) Relax completely on the back for 2 to 3 minutes.

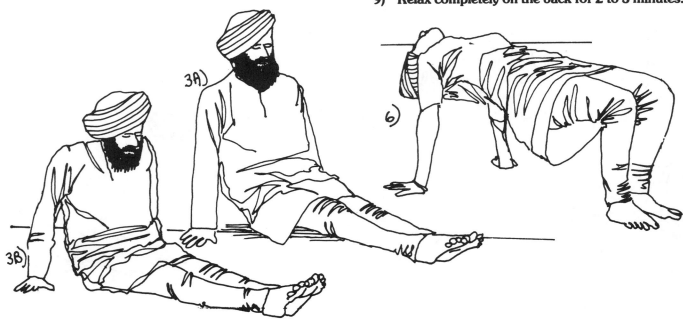

10) Come into bridge pose. Raise the right leg 60°. Point the toes forward. Do a powerful breath of fire for 1½ minutes. Then inhale deeply, exhale completely, and apply mul bhand. Repeat the exercise with the left leg raised. Relax.

11) Sit in crow pose. Squat down with the feet flat on the ground. With the palms facing down, extend the arms in front parallel to the ground. Inhale deeply as you stand up — exhale completely as you squat down. Keep the spine as straight as possible. Do 30 of these crow squats.

12) Lie on the stomach. Put the palms on the ground under the shoulders. Slowly arch up into cobra pose. Hold the pose with normal breathing for 1 minute. Then kick the buttocks with one leg for 2 minutes. Each time the heel strikes the buttocks, exhale slightly. Kick with the other leg for 2 more minutes. Relax.

13) Sit on the heels in rock pose. Extend the arms straight over the head with the palms flat together. Bring the palms down halfway toward the top of the head with the elbows slightly bent. Raise the eyes up and focus at the center of the skull on the pineal gland and through the top of the head. Continue for at least 3 minutes.

COMMENTS:

If sleep is a constant problem for you, practice this kriya regularly for 90 days. It can be done before bed at night or in the morning. We waste billions of dollars on sleeping aids and stimulants when a much safer and more stable approach exists in exercise and meditation. Unfortunately, the exercises take effort; a pill doesn't. If you choose to put the effort into this kriya, it will eliminate sleep disturbances and give you alertness throughout the day.

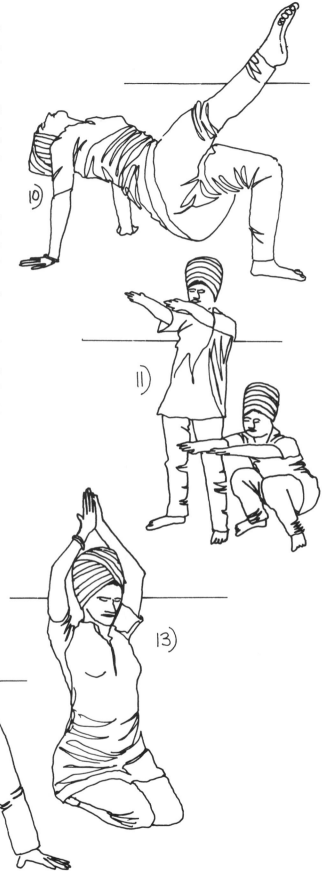

SITALI PRANAYAM

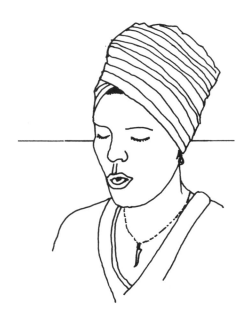

Sit in a comfortable meditative posture with the spine straight. Curl the tongue and protrude it slightly past the lips. Inhale deeply and smoothly through the tongue and mouth. Exhale through the nose. Continue for 5 minutes. Then inhale — hold. Pull in the tongue. Exhale and relax. Repeat this for two more 5-minute periods.

COMMENTS:

Sitali pranayam is a well known practice. It soothes and cools the spine in the area of the fourth, fifth, and sixth vertebrae. This, in turn, regulates the sexual and digestive energy. This breath is often used for lowering fever. Great powers of rejuvenation and detoxification are attributed to this breath when practiced regularly. Doing 52 breaths daily can extend your lifespan. Often the tongue may taste bitter at first. This is a sign of toxification. As you continue the practice the taste of the tongue will ultimately become sweet.

EXERCISES TO MAKE THE PORES BREATHE

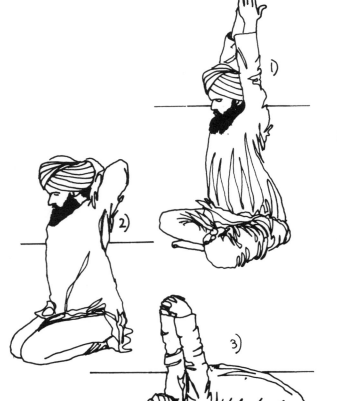

1) Sit in easy pose. Place the palms together overhead with arms straight hugging the ears. Begin breath of fire and continue for 2 minutes. Inhale — hold for 20 seconds, exhale. Repeat breath of fire for 2 minutes. Inhale — hold 30 seconds, exhale. Repeat one more time. Relax for 2 minutes.

2) Sit on the heels in vajrasana (rock pose). Cross the hands behind the head and hold onto the shoulders with opposite hands. Begin breath of fire and continue for 2 minutes. Inhale — hold. Exhale — relax. Repeat breath of fire 1 minute, then relax 3 minutes.

3) Yoga mudra: Sit on the heels. Place the hands in venus lock behind the back. Lean forward and gradually bring the forehead to the ground. Raise the arms straight up to 90°, maintaining the position to maximum ability. Hold for at least 3 minutes.

4) Relax completely on the back for 10 minutes.

COMMENTS:

The skin breathes. It is just as important to keep its channels clean as it is for the nose or lungs. This series removes obstructions to the flow of prana through the "third lung."

PRANAYAM FOR PURIFICATION

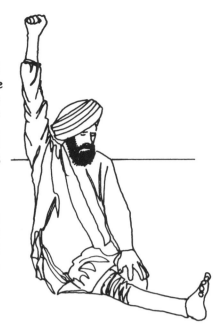

Sit on the left heel with the right leg extended forward. Stretch the right arm straight up and make a fist. Take long deep breaths, but try to squeeze the breath through the right nostril. Mentally vibrate *"Sat"* with the inhale and *"Nam"* with the exhale. Continue for 3 minutes. Then switch legs, arms, and nostrils. Begin a deep, powerful breath again for 3 minutes.

COMMENTS:

This breathing kriya is to eliminate negativity and the urge to slander others rather than purify yourself. It stimulates the lymphatic system to clean itself. It increases nerve energy in the entire body.

EXERCISES FOR EXPANDING LUNG CAPACITY

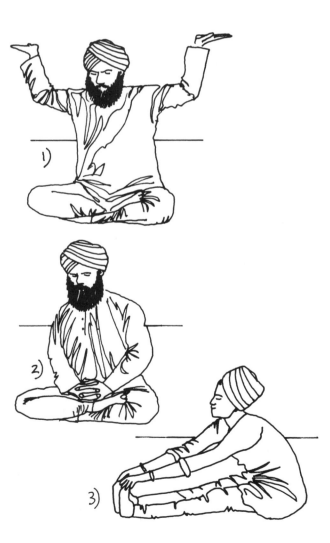

1) Sit in easy pose. Raise the arms up so that the upper arms are parallel to the ground and the forearms are perpendicular to the ground. Bend the wrists so that the palms are facing upward, parallel to the ground. Maintain this position for 1 minute. Inhale deeply and hold for 10 seconds. Exhale. Repeat the breaths without rest 4 times. Then hold the breath out and apply mul bhand. Inhale, hold briefly and exhale.

2) Do long deep breathing for 10 minutes with the hands in venus lock in the lap (2). With each inhalation, raise the rib cage up high. Temporary dizziness may be experienced, but the results will lead to mind control. Firm concentration at the brow will alleviate most imbalances.

3) This exercise must immediately follow the one above. Sit up with the legs straight out in front. Bend forward and hold the toes. Inhale, exhale and hold the breath out. Pump the belly as long as possible, then inhale and exhale. Repeat 2 more times.

COMMENTS:

Exercise 1 turns on the energy to the lungs and heart. Exercise 2 uses the energy to expand the lung capacity. Exercise 3 balances and distributes the prana. For a beginners' class, do this set 3 times, but allow only 2 - 3 minutes of breathing in exercise 2.

BASIC BREATH SERIES

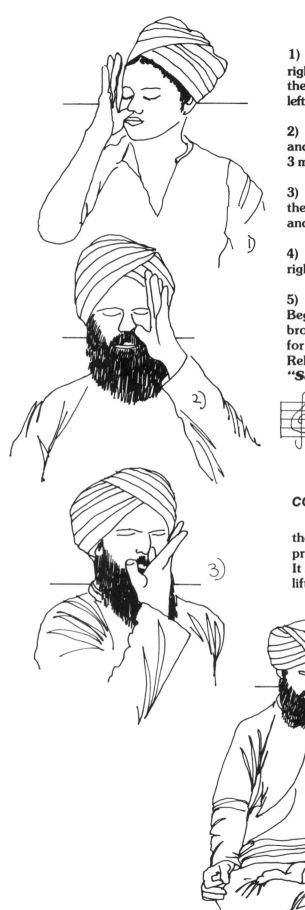

1) Sit in easy pose. Make an antenna of the right-hand fingers and block the right nostril with the thumb. Begin long deep breathing through the left nostril for 3 minutes. Inhale — hold for 10 seconds.

2) Repeat the first exercise, but use the left hand and breathe through the right nostril. Continue for 3 minutes. Inhale — hold for 10 seconds.

3) Inhale through the left nostril, exhale through the right using long deep breaths. Use the forefinger and little finger to close alternate nostrils.

4) Repeat exercise 3 except inhale through the right nostril and exhale through the left.

5) Sit in easy pose with hands in gyan mudra. Begin breath of fire. Totally center yourself at the brow point. Continue with a regular powerful breath for 7½ minutes. Then inhale, circulating the energy. Relax or meditate for 5 minutes, then chant long **"Sat Nam."**

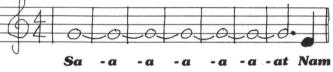

Sa -a -a -a -a -a -at Nam

COMMENTS:

This set opens the pranic channels and balances the breath in the two sides of your body. It is often practiced before a more strenuous, physical kriya. It is great to do by itself whenever you need a quick lift and a clear mind.

PRANAYAM SERIES

Pranayam Series #1

1) Sit in easy pose, the hands in gyan mudra with the arms straight. Begin breath of fire and continue for 7 minutes. Inhale — hold the breath for 30 seconds, exhale.

2) Begin long deep breathing through both nostrils. Breathe deeper than normal so that the entire rib cage lifts several inches. Continue 5 minutes, then inhale — hold 15 seconds, exhale.

3) Immediately begin to breathe in through puckered lips and exhale through the nose. Continue 3 minutes. Then inhale — hold briefly, exhale.

4) Do a powerful and regular breath of fire for 2 minutes. Then inhale deeply — hold as long as is comfortable. Focus at the brow point.

5) Meditate with normal breathing. Feel the flow of energy through the whole body.

Pranayam Series #2

Sit in easy pose, hands in gyan mudra. Make a "U" out of the right hand. Inhale through the left nostril holding the right one shut with the thumb (A). Exhale out the right nostril holding the left one shut with the little finger (B). Think **"Sat"** on the inhale and **"Nam"** on the exhale. Continue for 10 minutes with deep, regular breaths. Then inhale, exhale, inhale, exhale completely and hold it out. Apply the mul bhand.

COMMENTS:

The first kriya is a good blood cleanser and energizer. The second is for emotional balance. If you get up some morning and feel that you "got up on the wrong side of bed," this exercise will rebalance you for the day.

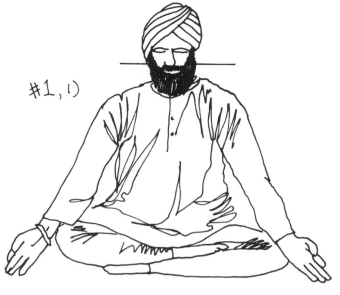

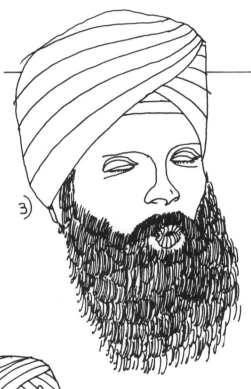

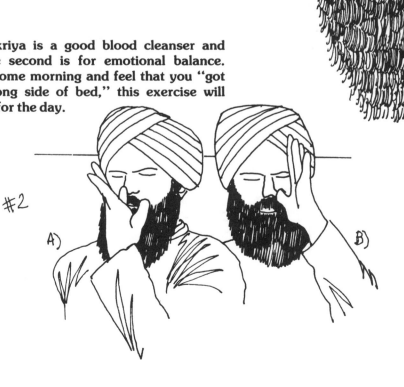

BEGINNERS EXERCISE I

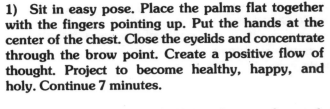

1) Sit in easy pose. Place the palms flat together with the fingers pointing up. Put the hands at the center of the chest. Close the eyelids and concentrate through the brow point. Create a positive flow of thought. Project to become healthy, happy, and holy. Continue 7 minutes.

2) Lie down on the back. Point the toes forward. Begin long deep breaths for 5 minutes. Then relax for 2 minutes.

3) Still lying on the back, begin breath of fire for 1 minute, then inhale and hold for 15 seconds. Take 8 long, deep, complete breaths. Repeat this entire sequence 3 times.

4) Relax for 2 minutes.

5) Lie on the back. Point the toes forward. Lift both legs 6 inches off the ground as you inhale deeply. Hold the position for 15 seconds. Lower the legs. Repeat this 5 times.

6) Deeply relax the body part by part for 10 minutes.

COMMENTS:

This is an easy set to practice for beginners. The effect of the breath is to open the lungs and diaphragm and to slightly stimulate the navel center. The stimulation of these two energy resources allows a deep relaxation. This set is excellent for releasing a normal day's tension build-up.

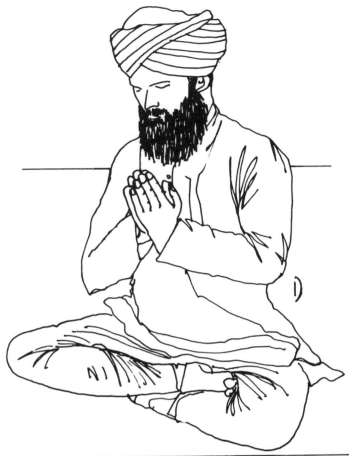

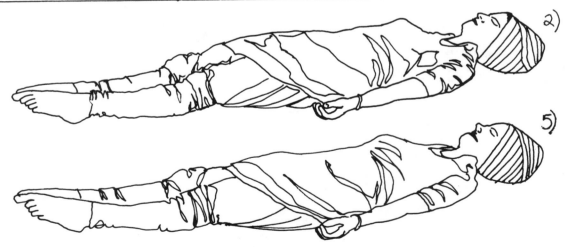

BEGINNERS EXERCISE II

Sit on the left heel. Extend the right leg forward and point the toes. Bend forward and grasp the right toes with both hands. Keep the spine as straight as you can and look toward the toes. Hold this position for 2 minutes, then begin breath of fire for 1 minute. Switch legs and repeat the exercise. Relax for 1 minute.

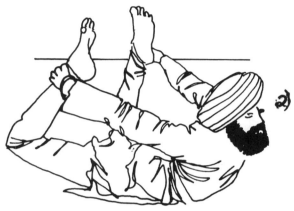

2) Lie on the stomach. Grab the ankles and stretch up like a bow. Do breath of fire for 2 minutes. Then relax down.

3) Sit between the heels (celibate pose). Raise the arms up at a 60° angle to the horizontal with the palms facing each other. Bounce up and down with the breath. Inhale as you raise up and exhale as you drop down. After 1 minute, exhale deeply. Hold the breath out and apply mul bhand. Repeat one more time.

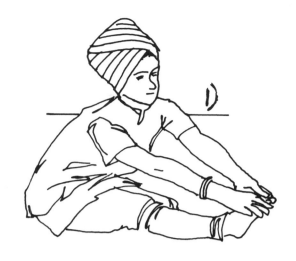

4) Stand up. Stretch up on toes. Raise the arms straight up. Stretch up. Then bounce up and down for five seconds. Then sit down in easy pose. Slowly come up without using the hands. Continue to repeat the exercise cycle for 2 minutes.

5) Sit in an easy posture. Put the hands in gyan mudra. Go deep within for 5 minutes.

COMMENTS:

This kriya transforms sexual energy into meditative energy. It strengthens the nerves in the upper thighs that regulate sexual potency. Exercises 1 and 2 release the Kundalini energy for self-healing. Repeat the kriya 2 to 3 times for a more advanced workout that will make sweat.

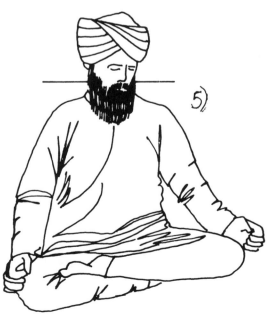

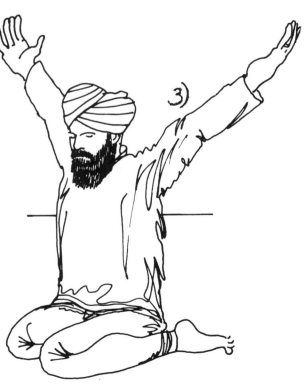

PREPARATORY EXERCISES FOR LUNGS, MAGNETIC FIELD AND DEEP MEDITATION

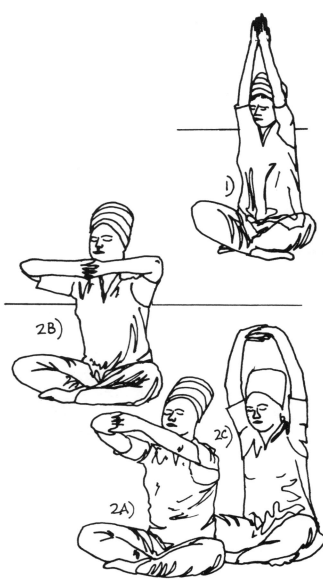

1) Sit in easy pose. Stretch the arms straight up overhead with palms together. Arch the spine as far up and back as possible. Begin long deep breathing through the mouth with a whistle both on the inhale and the exhale. Continue this for 5 minutes. Relax.

2) Stretch the arms straight out in front, fingers interlocking with the palms facing outward (2A). Exhale, bring the hands in towards the chest (2B). Inhale, stretch the arms out straight again. Continue for 2 minutes with a fairly rapid motion. Then inhale, stretch the arms out straight in front, the fingers interlocking, with the palms facing outward (2A). Hold the breath and bring the arms straight up over the head (2C). Bring them back down parallel to the floor (2A). Exhale and bring the hands in toward the chest (2B). Inhale, stretch the arms out straight in front again, and repeat the sequence for 2 minutes.

3) Without resting, stretch the arms out straight in front at a 60° angle to each other. Inhale - slowly clench the fists. Hold the breath and, with tension, bring the fists to the chest, bending the arms at the elbows. Exhale — release the tension. Repeat for 3 minutes, maintaining an angry face throughout the exercise.

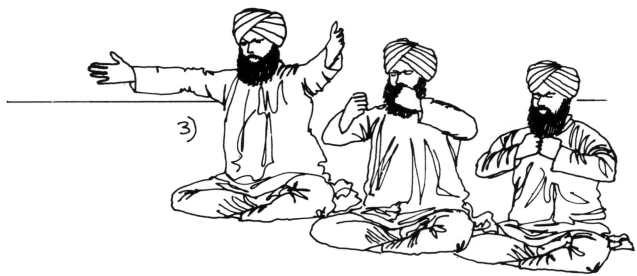

4) Place the hands with fingers interlocked and palms facing upward behind the neck (4A). Inhale — stretch arms up overhead (4B). Exhale down behind the neck. Continue for 2 minutes.

5) Stretch the arms straight up overhead, palms together, thumbs crossed. Inhale and twist to the left. Exhale and twist right. Continue for 2 minutes.

6) Interlock the fingers at chest level, with palms facing down (6A). Inhale, bring the hands up to eye level (6B). Exhale back down to chest level. Continue for 2 minutes.

7) Place the hands on shoulders, fingers in front, thumbs in back. Inhale — twist to the left. Exhale — twist to the right. Continue for 2 minutes.

8) Sit in easy pose. Place the hands on knees (8A). Inhale — flex both shoulders up (8B). Exhale down. Continue for 2 minutes. Then begin to flex the spine. Inhale forward, exhale back. Continue for 2 minutes.

9) Roll the eyes up as far as possible. Concentrate at the top of the head. Meditate for 15 minutes.

COMMENTS:

This series begins by purifying the blood and expanding the lung capacity. Then the circulatory system is stimulated. The thyroid and parathyroid secretions are added to the increased circulation and the upper magnetic field of the body is enlarged. This is an excellent preparation for beginners who need to learn deep meditation.

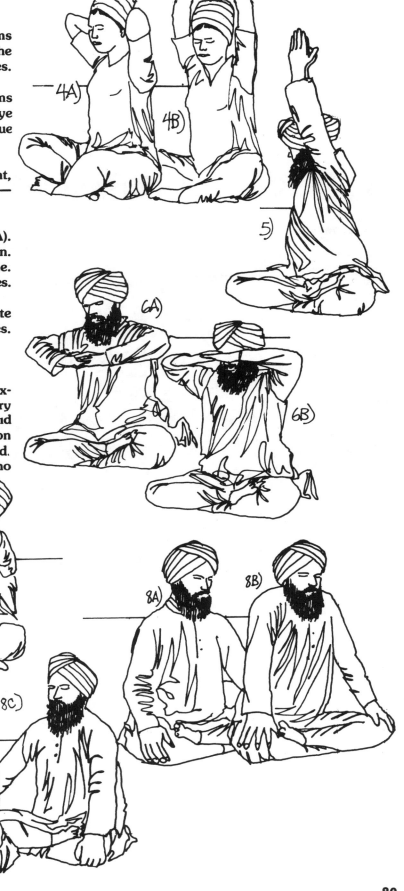

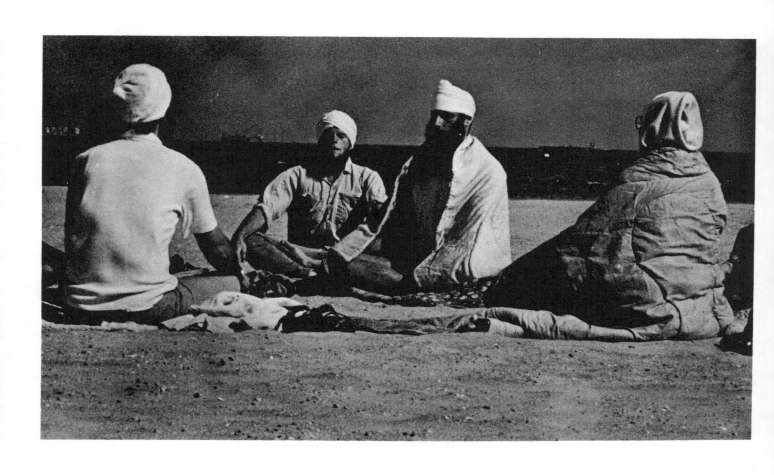

Creative Meditation

Individual / Universal Harmony

By Siri Singh Sahib Bhai Sahib

Harbhajan Singh Khalsa Yogiji

These days there is a trend toward meditation in America, Western Europe and many other countries, but there is also much misunderstanding. I would like to go into the depth of the subject. Our job is to teach it through the universities and to teach you what is what so that you can know the nature of what you are asking for. Then you can practice any way you like. Does anybody know what meditation is?

Audience Response: "It would be like a silencing of the mind from everyday life and allowing the free flow of thought."

Audience Response: "It is concentration."

That's part of it. Anybody else?

Audience Response: "It is complete relaxation from regular hassles."

Come on, come on, everybody.

Audience Response: "It's a new level of consciousness, a deeper level of consciousness. It's not exactly the same thing as our state of consciousness when we're doing something or when we have to relate to some function."

Audience Response: "It is becoming receptive."

You all have one part or the other of meditation. Prayer is when the mind is one-pointed and man talks to infinity. Meditation is when the mind becomes totally clean and receptive and infinity talks to man. That is what meditation is. There are two levels of meditation. In one, this unit self talks to infinity. In the other, infinity talks to the unit. All the other stages are preparations for meditation.

You might have heard alot these days about transcendental meditation and integral meditation and so many other meditations. If you want to sell mustard seed, you may call it yellow mustard, sun valley mustard seed, California mustard seed, Wisconsin mustard seed, or New York mustard seed; but the mustard seed is still a mustard seed. Meditation was labeled with many different names. Similarly in yoga, the techniques to raise the Kundalini were all different, but they were given different names. Hatha yoga has the same end, which is to raise the Kundalini in a person. Raja yoga also has the same end. Bhakti, Shakti, Gyan, Karma yoga — they all have the same end: they all want to raise the dormant power of infinity in

man. That's all. There is a small difference. Suppose you want to go to San Francisco. You can take Highway 1 or 5 or an aircraft or a railway line or go on a truck or hitchhike. The purpose is to reach San Francisco. By foot you can make it in two months or a month or twenty days; hitchhiking takes two days; a railway line takes one or two days; a car takes eight or ten hours; an aircraft will take you 45 minutes. Highway 1 will take you ten hours; Highway 5 will take you six and a half hours. It is true that man has an infinite power which he can connect with through the techniques of yoga. There are different yogas around, different ways to go. Some take thirty years to practice while others take thirty days. The difference is only in time and technique.

The best way to meditate is in a creative meditation. The logic behind this is that the mind is mostly tuned to the intellect. The intellect starts giving thoughts and more thoughts, of which relate to your emotion and temperament. They become desires, and desire then directs the body to create a creativity to earn the object or goal. This creativity is a practical experience in life.

Once I decided to rent a building. My staff said, "No, we want to have a permanent address. We don't want to rent. We will have to move, then later we will have to move again, etc." God sent us a person who found this property on Preuss Road, so I bought it. Once we bought it, everything went into it. We creatively thought about it and acted on it. Our one concern became, "What is the best atmosphere, what are the best circumstances, and in what way are they creative?" We put our whole energy into it in a very well-balanced manner. The result is this creative place and atmosphere we are teaching in tonight.

You can't live without meditation. Imagination and activity get blended to affect the focusing of the personality. That's what meditation is. You relate your unit activity towards your word of infinity. The question is: Are you creative or uncreative? That will decide the trend of your life. If you just sit for twenty minutes and close yourself that's not meditation. That is an effort, and attempt to prepare yourself for meditation. It is a preparation, not a complete result. Meditation is the creativity and activity which relates your existence to the existence of the cosmos. It is individual harmony in relationship to universal harmony.

When you come into contact with a living identity and remember infinity — that is God. When you meet a good man and you feel fulfilled — that is divine. Whenever you meet a living existence that enables you to expand to infinity in consciousness, you experience God. God is not a man. God is three letters, G—O—D, that represent the generating principle, the organizing principle, and the destroying principle. They took the first letter from each of those three words and made one word: GOD. The Hindus speak of Brahma, the god who gives birth; Vishnu, the god who sustains; and Shiva, the god who destroys. The Hindus whorship them in idols. We have one word, GOD, which represents the same thing.

All churches and temples, synagogues and holy palces are holy because the whole community can get together and relate together in unity unto infinity. That is why they are beautiful. Otherwise they have no purpose. They are places of creativity through divine meditation.

Audience Response: "Well I get confused when you say..."

First of all remember that when you say, "I get confused," you are creating a vibration which confuses you. Don't use negative words. That is an uncreative meditation through a creative faculty. Three phrases you should never use: "I am confused," "I don't know," "I can't do it."

There are two parallel tendencies in a person: the urge to suicide and the urge to live. The higher mind runs on the living tendencies and does not go along with the suicidal tendencies. I feel it is my right to live because I have been created by the infinity that is a Creator. Which tendency prevails depends on which you choose through your meditation and your words. Without creative meditation, a man will feel burdened. The law of detachment does not become functional for a man if he is not creative. Remember this law. It is the secret of spirituality which I'm explaining. Creative meditation is meditation in activity which links you with infinity.

Detachment does not mean that you wear a loin cloth and carry a begging bowl and are detached from this world. Detachment comes from creative activity. If you only create a few things, you will feel attached to them. If you are constantly creating, you will feel free. You have been involved in many affairs and you have learned about failure and success. This has brought you to a state of attachment which will limit you. God has not made any person to limit himself. Man is not born to be limited. Death and life mean nothing to those who live moment to moment in happiness, joy and creativity.

Audience Response: "Can you be detached from your own emotions?"

Why should you be detached from your emo-

tions? You don't have to get rid of emotions and you don't have to have them either. You can just watch them. Let the emotion come. Let emotion go. What comes should go. It is not emotions which prove that you're alive. The way to find that out is to check your nose. If the breath goes in and out, then you are still alive.

You want to feel, I know. But has it ever occurred to you that you are so beautiful that the whole universe wants to tell you? Once you realize that you are invaluable, you don't have to make value judgements. Values come from attachment. We put a price on each other because of our limited self; otherwise, each one is priceless. Where is the limit of a person? His limit is in his attachment. Man is basically unlimited because his soul is unlimited. Man is basically unlimited because his mind is unlimited. This structure is limited but it is priceless. Nobody can manufacture anything like this. Creative meditation uses this structure in relation to the cosmos.

Do you know how things go on around this earth? Science may find within a thousand years that the life-sound comes from the sun. That sound is the existence of the atom. Then they will find that we have within us a little sun. Therefore our existence is also the existence of the atom, and we make an impact on the universe just as it makes an impact on us. Every person thinks he knows everything without knowing what he knows. That is the mystery of life. We all know how successful we can be without knowing what success is. Does anybody know what success is?

Audience Response: "The opposite of failure."

That is the right answer. You think that riches make you successful? I can give you telephone numbers of rich people who have got plenty of money and comfort. All they want is to be able to sleep. If you think power is success, I can also give you the numbers of powerful people. They think they are God if they can get time to eat or relax. It is a strange, strange world. I have everything which a normal American can think of, but I am still free.

We get so attached to things! If it is the rainy season, we get upset, as if we were paper and were going to melt. If it is summer, we get upset. If there were no summer, what would happen? Somebody was saying to me, "Oh, spring is coming. There will be hayfever." The moment spring comes people start thinking of hayfever. Nobody thinks of the beauty of spring when everything blooms.

When your mind is totally creative, nothing will come to you without a purpose. Nothing will happen to you without a purpose. Nothing will bind you with attachment to the cycle of worry and pain. Success will be a subconscious habit. Creative meditation is when the creative mind accepts itself as part of the universe. The whole universe then be comes part of you. A creative mind knows that wherever he is he can be creative. When you become a part of the universe, the universe becomes part of you. That is creative meditation — minute to minute, time to time, being to being, place to place, and breath to breath. Each breath which goes in you goes in under the divine will and it comes out under divine will. So what are you worried about?

Who among you has the power to breathe? What is breath to you? It means life. It is life. What is life? Life is a *bindu*, a point. It has been vitalized and energized to go in the longitude and latitude on the orbit of time to a specific length. Its glow depends on its own vibration. If your vibration is universal, you've become a universal man. If it's national, you've become a national man. If you have a city vibration, you are a city man. If you are little, you are a little man. You can decide. That much is your choice. As you expand your mind, you expand. As you limit your mind, you are limited.

Life is not under your control and the mind is not obedient, but there is something the mind does obey. That is the rate of the breath. The mind knows if its body is not going to have breath, the mind will have nothing to do with the body. When the breath is long and deep and slow, the mind is constant and one-pointed. When the breath is heavy, quick, and shallow, the mind is scattered. You normally breathe 15 breaths a minute. If you can train yourself to breathe eight breaths per minute, you can have your temper and your projection under control. It is the most creative meditation you can do. Expand the mind and become part of the whole cosmic process. Become creative, unattached, and carefree, but not careless. Take meditation to heart as a golden path to infinity which must be experienced in practical activity each day.

MEDITATIONS

LAYA YOGA MEDITATION

1) Sit in easy pose with a straight spine. Take your right thumb and block off the right nostril. Begin deep breathing through the left nostril. Close the eyes and survey the body up and down ten deep breaths through the left nostril, following with ten deep breaths through the right nostril. Continue for 2 minutes.

2) Put palms together and bring them to the chest about the level of the heart, three inches above the sternum. Apply a slight pressure to the middle of the chest. Begin long deep breathing for 2 minutes; then breath of fire for 1 minute.

3) Put the hands in gyan mudra and the arms at 60° and do long deep breathing for 2 minutes.

4) Keeping the hands in gyan mudra, lower the arms, resting the wrists on the knees with the elbows straight. Begin the 3½-cycle spin chant, pulling mul bhand. With the breath, spin the sound current up the spine. Let go and get lost in the spin. Visualize the sound spinning from the base of the spine to the top of the head. Use the Adi Shakti Mantra: *"Ek Ong Kar-a, Sat-a Nam-a, Siri Wha-a He Guru."* On *"Ek,"* pull the navel point. On *"a,"* the diaphragm lock (*uddiyana bhand).* On *"He Guru,"* relax the lock. Continue from 11 to 31 minutes.

COMMENTS:

There are two voices within us: One is the voice of the ego and the other, the voice of the soul. Justify yourself before the Creator, not before others. Consciously remember the link between you and your Creator.

If you can keep away from negativity, you are a living god on this earth. This meditation enables one to get lost in the sound current. "Meditate and feel God for 40 days and you will be liberated."

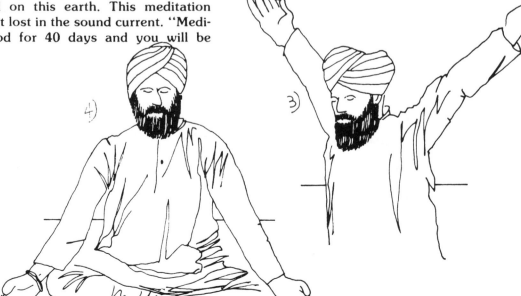

SEVEN-WAVE "SAT NAM" MEDITATION

Sit in easy pose. Place the palms flat together at the center of the chest, thumbs touching the center of the sternum. With the eyes closed, look up slightly, focusing at the brow point. Inhale deeply, concentrating on the breath. With the exhale, chant the mantra in the law of seven or law of the tides. Vibrate *"Sat"* in six waves, and let *"Nam"* be the seventh.

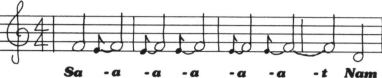

Sa -a -a -a -a -a -t Nam

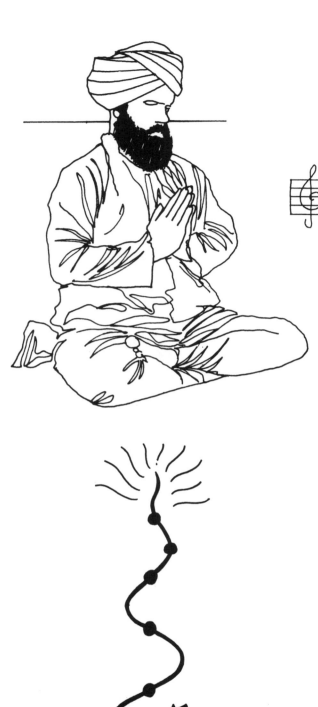

On each wave, thread the sound through the chakras beginning at the base of the spine in the rectum. On *"Nam,"* let the energy and sound radiate from the seventh chakra at the top of the head through the aura. As the sound penetrates each chakra, or center, gently pull the physical area it corresponds to. The first center is the rectum, the second is the sex organs, the third is the navel point, the fourth is the heart, the fifth is the throat, the sixth is the brow point and the seventh is the top of the head. Continue for 15 minutes.

COMMENTS:

If you can build this meditation to at least 31 minutes 6 seconds per day, the mind will be cleansed as the ocean waves wash the sandy beach.

This is a *bij* (seed) mantra meditation. Bij mantras such as *"Sat Nam"* are the only sounds which can totally rearrange the habit patterns of the subconscious mind. We all have habit patterns. We could not function without them, but sometimes the patterns we have created are not wanted. You have changed, so you want the patterns to change. By vibrating the sound current *"Sat Nam"* in this manner, you activate the energy of the mind that erases and establishes habits. Consequently, this meditation is good to do as an introduction to Kundalini yoga. It will open the mind to new experience. A long-time student will still meditate in this way, particularly to clear off the effects of a hurried day before beginning another deep meditation. After you chant this mantra, you will feel calm, relaxed and mellow.

RAJA YOGA MEDITATION WITH MAHA BHAND

1) Sit in any easy sitting posture. The spine must be perfectly straight. Rest both hands gently in the lap (1A). For a female, the left hand rests on top of the right. For the male, it is reversed (1B). Close the eyes and concentrate at the brow point. Focus the attention at the tip of the big toe and mentally draw the life force along the entire length of the leg to the rectum and rotate the energy around the ring of the rectum. Inhale deeply — pull the rectum up, then release it. Continue rhythmical pulling and then exhale. Repeat the cycle, inhaling from toe to rectum Each time try to pull the rectum further up.

2) Inhale and pull the sex organ as well as the rectum. Contract it and pull up 5 times per breath.

3) Pull the navel point, sex organ and rectum 5 times per breath. Try to massage the spine with the navel point. Pull the lower triangle further up each time until the energy is pulled all the way to the diaphragm.

4) Inhale deeply and concentrate on the Divine Power in the breath. Feel it shoot up to the diaphragm like a rocket as the locks are pulled. Lift up the chest to lift the diaphragm. Exhale.

5) Inhale — pull all the locks and pull the chin in to form the neck lock, or *jalandhara bhand*, concentrate on consciously raising the energy to the neck. A heat will be created there.

6) Inhale — pull the energy all the way to the brow point. Apply all the lower locks and press the eyes up. Exhale.

7) Relax, meditate at the brow, and go deep within.

8) Meditate at the brow point, and chant very sweetly from the back of your throat at the upper palate of the mouth:

LA - a - a - a - a - a - a - ah

Create a continuous sound, inhaling when necessary. Listen to the sound as though it comes from infinity. After 5 minutes, inhale deeply. Tilt the head back and look at the sky. Let the breath out with a laugh. Keep laughing aloud for 30 seconds. Relax.

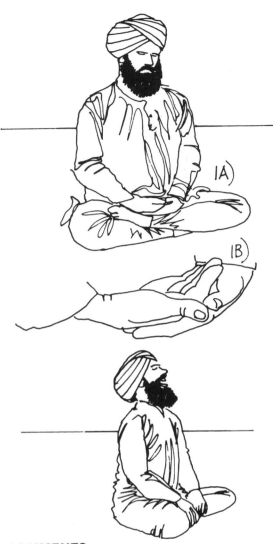

COMMENTS:

Parts 1 through 6 should be practiced 5 minutes each. Part 7, the final meditation, may be as long as you want. The chanting of *"Laaah"* may be extended to 11 minutes. It is best to practice this meditation ½ to 1 hour each day.

Raja yoga is a part of Kundalini yoga. There are many meditations in this part of the tradition. This meditation awakens the God in you. There is no need to find God. He already exists in you as Infinite Awareness. It is only necessary to awaken Him. This meditation can open the third eye and give you the practical experience of a reality which cannot be put into words. Raja yoga relates the mind directly to the soul or self. So, there is no automatic control over the mind except will. Kundalini yoga generally relates the body directly to soul so that the mind has no option but to follow the will to infinity.

This series will automatically relate your circumvent force to the universal magnetic field. The more you consciously invest your mind into this, the more expansion you will experience. The practice is self-styling and will direct your conscious energy.

KIRTAN KRIYA

Sit straight in easy pose (A). Meditate at the brow point and produce the five primal sounds, or the *Panj Shabad* — **S, T, N, M, A** — in the original word form:

SA — infinity, cosmos, beginning
TA — life, existence
NA — death
MA — rebirth

This is the cycle of creation. From the infinite comes life and individual existence. From life comes death or change. From death comes the rebirth of consciousness to the joy of the infinite through which compassion leads back to life. This sound current is represented musically this way:

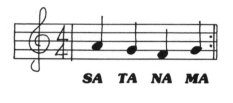

SA   TA   NA   MA

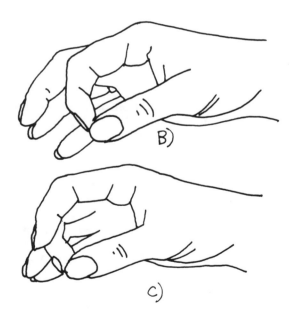

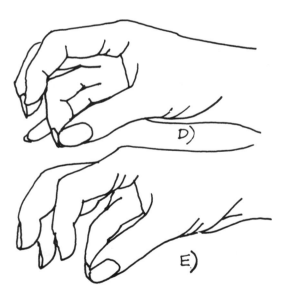

95

Each repetition of the entire mantra takes 3 to 4 seconds.

The elbows are straight while chanting, and each fingertip touches in turn the tip of the thumb with firm pressure.

On *"SA"* touch the first, the Jupiter finger, to the thumb (B).

On *"TA"* touch the second, the Saturn finger, to the thumb (C).

On *"NA"* touch the third, the Sun finger, to the thumb (D).

On *"MA"* touch the fourth, the Mercury finger, to the thumb (E).

Then begin again on the first finger.

Chant in the three languages of consciousness:

human — things, the world; normal or loud voice
lovers — longing to belong; strong whisper
divine — infinity; mentally (silent)

Begin the kriya in normal voice for 5 minutes, then whisper for 5 minutes and then go deep into the sound silently. Vibrate in silence for about 11 minutes, then come back to a whisper for 5 minutes, then aloud for 5 minutes.

To come completely out of the meditation, stretch the hands up as far as possible and spread them wide. Stretch the spine and take several deep breaths. Relax.

COMMENTS:

Each time you close a mudra by joining the thumb with a finger, your ego "seals" the effect of that mudra in your consciousness. The effects are as follows:

SIGN	FINGER	NAME	EFFECT
♃	1st	Gyan Mudra	*Knowledge*
♄	2nd	Shuni Mudra	*Wisdom, intelligence, patience*
☉	3rd	Surya Mudra	*Vitality—energy of life*
☿	4th	Budhi Mudra	*Ability to communicate*

Practicing this chant brings a total mental balance to the individual psyche. As you vibrate on each fingertip, you alternate your electrical polarities. The index and ring fingers are electrically negative, relative to the other fingers. This causes a balance in the electro-magnetic projection of the aura.

If during the silent part of the meditation your mind wanders uncontrollably, go back to a whisper, to a loud voice, to a whisper and back into silence. Do this as often as you need to.

Practicing this meditation is both a science and an art. It is an art in the way it molds consciousness and in the refinement of sensation and insight it produces. It is a science in the tested certainty of the results each technique produces. Meditations have coded actions to their reactions in the psyche. But because it is effective and exact it can also lead to problems *if not done properly.*

Some people may experience headaches from practicing Kirtan Kriya. The most common reason for this is improper circulation of prana in the solar centers. To avoid this problem or correct it if it has already occurred, you must meditate on the primal sounds in the "L" form. This means that when you meditate you feel there is a constant inflow of cosmic energy into your solar center, or tenth gate. As the energy enters the top chakra, you place Sa, Ta, Na, or Ma there. As you chant *"Sa,"* for example, the *"S"* starts at the top of your head and the *"A"* ends through the brow point as it is projected to infinity. This energy flow follows the energy pathway called the *golden cord* — the connection between the pineal and pituitary glands.

Chanting *"SA-TA-NA-MA"* is the primal or nuclear form of *"Sat Nam."* It has the energy of the atom in it since we are breaking the atom (or bij) of the sound, *"Sat Nam."*

You may use this chant in any position as long as you adhere to the following requirements:

1) Keep the spine straight.
2) Focus at the brow point.
3) Use the "L" form of meditation.
4) Vibrate the Panj Shabad in all three languages.
5) Use yogic common sense without fanaticism.

The Siri Singh Sahib said at the Winter Solstice of 1972 that a person who wears pure white and meditates on this sound current for 2½ hours a day for one year, will know the unknowable and see the unseeable. Through this constant practice, the mind awakens to the infinite capacity of the soul for sacrifice, service, and creation.

A TRANSCENDENTAL MEDITATION: MAHA SHAKTI CHALNEE INDRA MUDRA

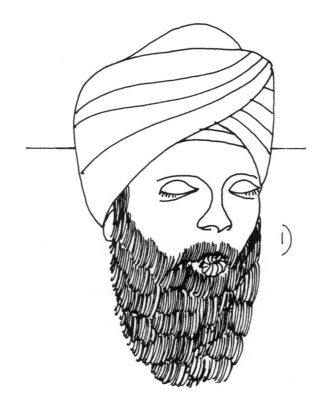

1) Sit in easy pose. Inhale with a deep whistle through the mouth. The lips should be puckered like a beak. Exhale through the nose. Concentrate the sound at the third eye point for 5 minutes. Listen just to the pure sound. Continue for 2 more minutes mentally inhaling *"Sat"* and exhaling *"Nam"* with the whistle.

2) Come into cobra pose. Arch the neck back and look up. Fix the eyesight at a point on the ceiling straight up. Inhale through the nose and whistle out through the mouth for 3 to 5 minutes. Inhale and slowly relax down out of cobra pose. Rest for 2 minutes.

3) Lie on the back with the knees pulled to the chest. Hold them there with hands and fingers interlaced over the knees. Lift the head up putting the nose between the knees. With the mouth *closed* make the sound *"hunnnnnnh."* The vibrations will be felt in the nose and throat. Continue for 3 minutes.

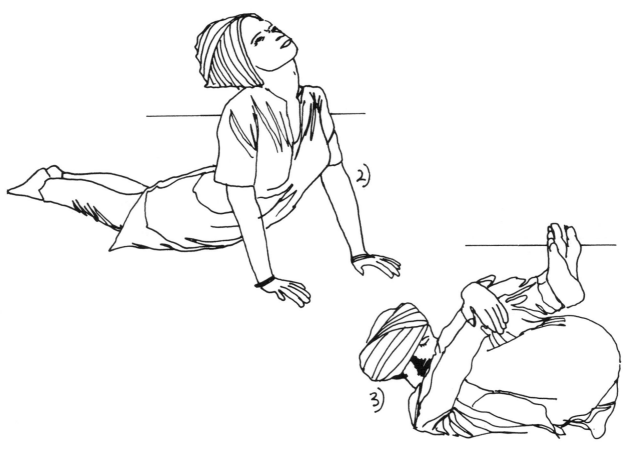

4) Relax on the back with legs crossed on the ground as in easy pose. This creates a delicate pressure in the lower spine. Maintain the position for 5 minutes.

5) Sit in easy pose, hands on the shoulders, thumbs behind and fingers in front. Swing from left to right, inhaling left and exhaling right (5A). Synchronize the motion with the breath for 1 minute. Then sit on the heels and continue the exercise for 1 more minute (5B). Inhale, hold briefly.

6) Still sitting on the heels, lean forward and put the forehead on the ground. Rest completely in this pose for 3 to 5 minutes.

COMMENTS:

This is a real transcendental meditation as it was originally taught centuries ago. If the many teachers who have come to the United States to initiate students into secret mantras claiming to be transcendental meditations actually gave the undiluted techniques like this kriya, then we would be able to research the science of consciousness much more effectively. Transcendental meditations always have a breath rhythm and a hand mudra linked to the mantra.

In the yogic scriptures, there are six pages written to tell the benefits of this single kriya. It allows you to control the senses and thoughts. It balances the life nerves of prana and apana so that your health is improved and the lung capacity is increased. Once your lung capacity for normal breathing goes beyond 700cc's, your personality changes. The extra capacity sends an increased vital force to the nervous system with each breath. Nerves that are strong give you patience. In this exercise, the body maintains a perfect equilibrium in the CO_2 and O_2 exchange. The pressure on the tongue causes the thyroid and parathyroids to secrete. If you practice part 1 for 15 minutes, you may experience some pain in the ears. After 31 minutes, you may have a pain in the upper chest. These are the signs of the glands secreting and gaining a new balance. If you sincerely practiced part 1 for 31 minutes a day followed by the remaining exercises, this kriya could change your personality, your total lifestyle, and even your destiny.

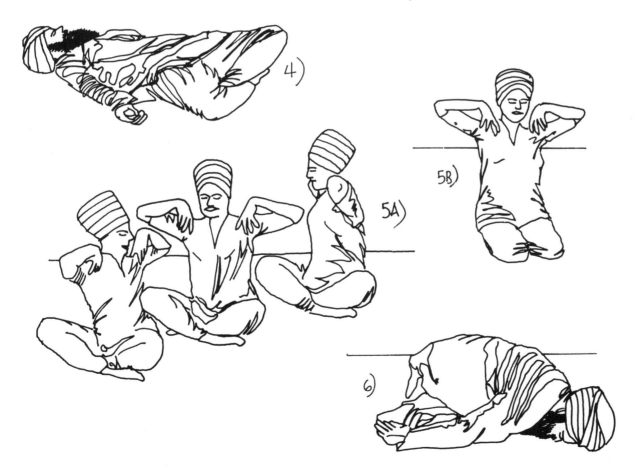

HEARTBEAT MEDITATION IN THE TRIPLE LOCK

Sit in easy pose or lotus pose with the hands in gyan mudra. The backs of the hands rest on the knees so the mudra faces upward (A). The touch of the fingers should be just hard enough to clearly feel your pulse in the tips of the thumbs.

The essence of this meditation is to form the triple lock in a relaxed, stable and attentive attitude. The *triple lock* is: 1) gyan mudra feeling your pulse, 2) front teeth locked on top of each other, tip to tip, 3) tongue turned backward as much as possible to touch the upper palate.

Meditate at the brow point on the constant rhythm of the heart. Keep the spine completely straight. Continue for 11 minutes. If you choose to practice this, slowly build the time each day until you can be alert for 31 minutes.

COMMENTS:

This meditation gives you the knowledge of past, present, and future. It directly activates the brain to associate new areas of the brain and balance the nervous system. If your spine is straight as you master this meditation, your entire destiny and self-concept will change and expand.

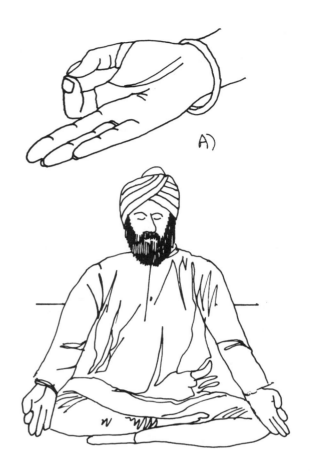

LAYA MEDITATION ON ECSTASY

Sit in easy pose keeping the arms straight with hands in gyan mudra resting on the knees. Sit very majestically as though in the court of a king. Close the eyes so that the energy of sight is not distracting from in-sight. Chant this laya mantra and enter a divine sound current. Concentrate and hear the sound within.

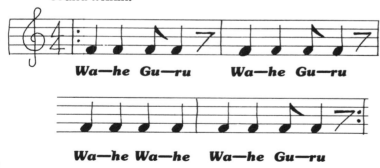

Wa—he Gu—ru   Wa—he Gu—ru

Wa—he Wa—he   Wa—he Gu—ru

Continue for 11 minutes, then inhale deeply and hold this precious breath. Concentrate the energy at the top of the head. After 30 seconds exhale and relax.

COMMENTS:

A fundamental motivation and instinct in man is to seek happiness. Usually we search all over the world for the right time, the right place, and the right partner, but we never find them all at one time, nor do any of them stay for long. Time, the great reaper, has its harvest of our sorrows and insecurities, but all we want is happiness.

A state of ecstasy exists within ourselves all the time. It is not dependent on the whims of circumstance and personality. It is an infinite pool that refreshes the heart and gives us strength to create a better self and a better world. This meditation leads you to that experience.

The mantra is a triple sound. As you continue the meditation it will lead your mind through three stages. The first stage is rhythmic and your mind will enjoy it, but it will still allow the thoughts of the day to enter. You will not like to put all your energy into ecstasy. In the second stage your self-conscious mind will reward you to feel yourself. This will happen because you will feel disturbed as your usual thoughts slip away. In the third stage you want to get rid of the self-consciousness and immerse yourself unconsciously into the ecstasy. You become so calm you want to sleep. It is the merging of a raindrop into a vastly calm and beautiful lake. You reflect all, cleanse all, refresh all. If you cross this third stage, you can know the ecstasy living within yourself and enter into a conscious balance and play with the Infinite.

MAHA AGNI PRANAYAM

Sit in easy pose or lotus position and place the palms together 9 to 12 inches in front of the chest at the level of the heart(A). Inhale and swing the head from the right shoulder across the chest to the left shoulder (B & C). Complete the swing by pulling the chin in facing straight forward (A). Focus at the brow point and project this mantra silently in perfect rhythm:

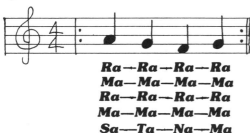

Ra—Ra—Ra—Ra
Ma—Ma—Ma—Ma
Ra—Ra—Ra—Ra
Ma—Ma—Ma—Ma
Sa—Ta—Na—Ma

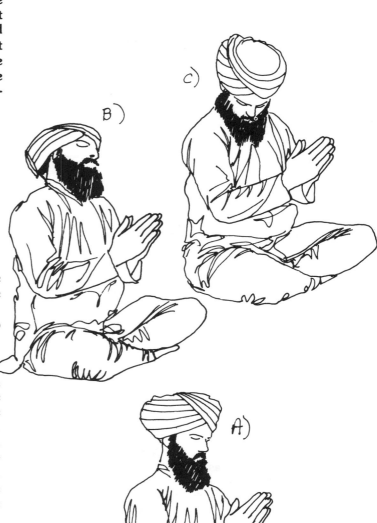

Exhale and immediately swing the head with the inhale. The head swing is quick and will give a little pull at the base of the skull.

Continue for 11 minutes and gradually build up the time to 31 minutes with practice.

COMMENTS:

This meditation can totally reorganize the brain secretions. In Kundalini yoga, the two halves of the brain are each divided into five main parts. The parts alternate in dominance every 2½ hours. During this kriya, the little fingers are touching from the base to the tip. This stimulates the heart meridian and connects the first and third brain areas, correlating your desires with what you achieve through action, and so you become a more effective being.

The head motion puts a pressure on the brain ducts to recirculate the spinal fluid into the blood stream. The circulation in the spinal fluid and meridians is often blocked at the base of the neck. This is particularly true of those who have used a drug like marijuana.

The sound of this mantra travels the mental orbit of your life. On **"RaRaRaRa MaMaMaMa RaRaRaRa MaMaMaMa,"** you travel from your central self into the orbit of mental life. **"Ra"** is the sun, **"Ma"** is the moon. You return with the bij mantra, **"Sa Ta Na Ma."** The rhythm is very important. If you cannot set the time of the mantra into a proper rhythm, the rhythm of the time cannot serve you. The moment you can reflect and create the proper rhythm of the time under the polarity of finite consciousness, then infinity has a right to serve you.

On the fourth and eleventh days of the moon cycle, there is a special pressure on the endocrine system to secrete and cleanse itself. To take advantage of this for your physical and mental health, practice this meditation for one hour on each of those days. The kriya will have the maximum value to you on these special days.

GURU GOBIND SINGH
SHAKTI MANTRA MEDITATION

Sit in easy pose with the elbows straight and hands in gyan mudra. Close the eyelids, concentrate at the brow point and chant two complete cycles of this mantra with each single breath:

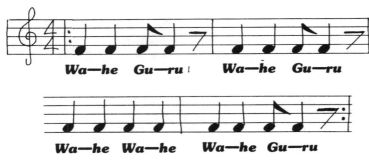

Wa—he Gu—ru   Wa—he Gu—ru

Wa—he Wa—he   Wa—he Gu—ru

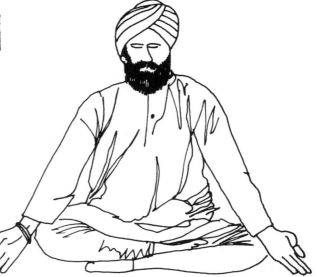

After chanting the two cycles, take a deep but rapid breath and repeat. A complete breath takes 12 seconds. Continue for 11 to 31 minutes. Inhale and concentrate the energy at the top of the head.

COMMENTS:

This is the science of Laya yoga. It is exact and exacting and it is nobody's private property. Those who have turned this into the secret possession of a few do a disservice to humanity at a time when people need every technique to grow. Laya yoga is a science of relating breath, rhythm and mantra to produce altered states of consciousness. Each *japa* (repetition of mantra) creates *tapa* (psychic heat). When you rotate the breath and volume of sound properly, it creates heat that burns off the karma. The knowledge cannot properly be transferred by secret whispering in the ears of disciples. It must be an open and conscious effort to expand your higher consciousness into practical expression. The relationship between your life in the finite and infinite depends on the rhythm of the breath. By controlling the breath, this kriya gives you a consciousness of ecstasy and calms the nerves. This calmness can also help to reduce fever.

MEDICAL MEDITATION FOR HABITUATION

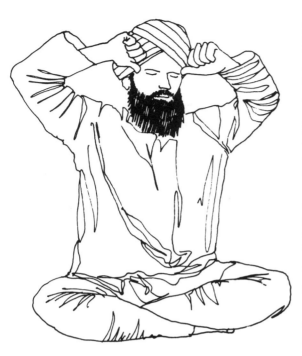

Sit in a comfortable pose. Straighten the spine and make sure the first six lower vertebrae are locked forward. Make fists of both hands and extend the thumbs straight. Place the thumbs on the temples and find the niche where the thumbs just fit. This is the lower anterior portion of the frontal bone above the temporal-sphenoidal suture.

Lock the back molars together and keep the lips closed. Vibrate the jaw muscles by alternating the pressure on the molars. A muscle will move in rhythm under the thumbs. Feel it massage the thumbs and apply a firm pressure with the hands.

Keep the eyes closed and look toward the center of the eyes at the brow point. Silently vibrate the five primal sounds, *"Sa Ta Na Ma,"* at the brow. Continue 5 to 7 minutes. With practice the time can be increased to 20 minutes and ultimately to 31 minutes.

COMMENTS:

This meditation is one of a class of meditations that will become well-known to the future medical society. Meditation will be used to alleviate all kinds of mental and physical afflictions, but it may be as many as 500 years before the new medical science will understand the effects of this kind of meditation well enough to delineate all its parameters in measurable factors.

The pressure exerted by the thumbs triggers a rhythmic reflex current into the central brain. This current activates the brain area directly underneath the stem of the pineal gland. It is an imbalance in this area that makes mental and physical addictions seemingly unbreakable.

In modern culture, the imbalance is pandemic. If we are not addicted to smoking, eating, drinking or drugs, then we are addicted subconsciously to acceptance, advancement, rejection, emotional love, etc. All these lead us to insecure and neurotic behavior patterns.

The imbalance in this pineal area upsets the radiance of the pineal gland itself. It is this pulsating radiance that regulates the pituitary gland. Since the pituitary regulates the rest of the glandular system, the entire body and mind go out of balance. This meditation corrects the problem. It is excellent for everyone but particularly effective for rehabilitation efforts in drug dependence, mental illness, and phobic conditions.

TAPA YOG KARAM KRIYA

Sit in a meditative pose. Extend the arms straight forward parallel to the ground. Palms face each other. Put the wrists together. Then spread the palms out as fas as you can as though pushing against a wall. The eyes are slightly open looking down at the tip of the nose. Begin rhythmically chanting: **Sat Nam, Sat Nam, Sat Nam, Sat Nam, Sat Nam, Sat Nam, Wahe Guru.** Continue for 11 minutes.

COMMENTS:

We cannot improve the caliber of the human being, but we can guide it. When we guide ourselves and are not at the mercy of subconscious habits then we become master of the self. But overcoming old habits and starting new ones requires strong nerves and willpower. This kriya develops willpower and gives the capacity to understand the elements of your personality. You can know what you are thinking and regulate the flow of those thoughts. This kriya is a perfect sadhana for difficulty in completing projects and doing what you intend.

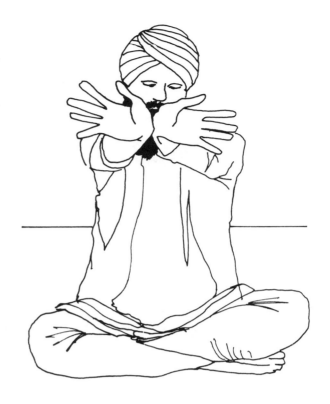

MEDITATION FOR THE LOWER TRIANGLE

Sit in easy pose. Make sure the spine is pulled up and stretched straight. Extend the right arm straight up hugging the ear. Extend the left arm to 60° from horizontal, with the palm facing down. On both hands, put the thumb onto the mound just below the little finger. Keep the eyes slightly open. Look down toward the upper lip. Press the elbows straight. Stretch the arms up from the shoulders. Continue for 11 minutes.

COMMENTS:

This meditation alleviates any problem in the lower spine. It is a direct healer for the kidneys and adrenal glands. Consequently it helps repair the energy drained by long term stress. This kriya also helps the heart. Although there is no breath specified, the breath will automatically become longer and deeper as you continue. It is important to hold the arms perfectly still to receive the full benefit.

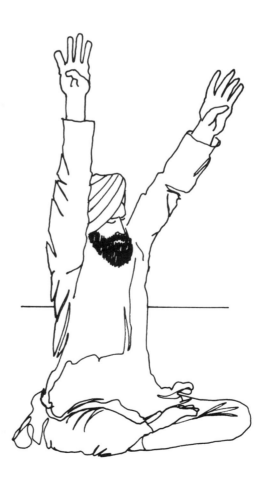

MEDITATION FOR BROSA

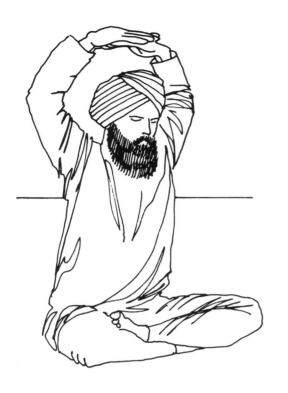

Sit in lotus or easy pose. Arch the arms up over the head with the palms down. If you are a male, put the right palm on top of the left. Ladies put the left palm on top of the right. Put the thumbtips together with thumbs pointing back. The arms are bent at the elbows slightly. Keep the eyelids open slightly and look down toward the upper lip.

Chant the mantra **Wahe Guru.** Form the sounds with the lips and tongue very precisely. Whisper it so that the **Guru** is almost inaudible. It takes about 2½ seconds per repetition. Continue for 11 minutes.

COMMENTS:

This kriya is very potent and must be respected. When beginning to experience this meditation, it should be done for a maximum of 11 minutes. Then increase the time by 1 minute after every 15 days of practice until you reach a total of 31 minutes. The effects are extensive. The meditation affects the element of trust in the human personality. Trust is the basis of faith and commitment and the sense of reality. It will give you the elevation of spirit so you can stand up to any challenge. It builds and balances the aura from the fourth chakra up.

MEDITATION FOR HUMAN QUALITY

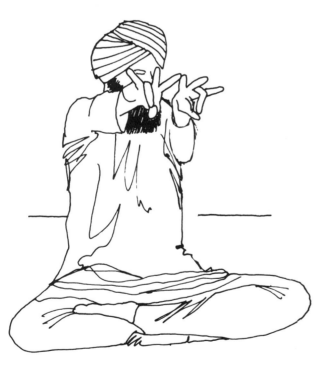

Sit in an easy cross-legged pose, keeping the spine straight. With both hands form Ravi mudra: Touch the tip of the ring finger to the tip of the thumb. Extend both arms parallel to the ground with the palms down. Spread the fingers wide. Put the sides of the tips of the index fingers together. Raise the arms slightly so the index fingernails are at the level of the eyes. Keep the eyes relaxed and open. Look over the index fingertips to the horizon. Just hold this position completely still. Continue for a maximum of 11 minutes.

COMMENTS:

We often fail in life and in our capacity for devotion because we are not trained to use our human qualities. These qualities of endurance, creativity, and compassion are regulated by the third, fourth and fifth chakras. The first and second chakras are below human. The sixth, seventh and eighth chakras are *beyond* human. So it is only in the area of the heart that we can fulfill our nature. This meditation opens the power of the fourth chakra. It balances and repairs the sympathetic nervous system. It helps the physical heart. It gives resistance to tension and high pressure environments. The greatest result is that it connects you with the inner sense of being human.

WHA GURU KRIYA
FOR NERVOUS BALANCE

Sit in lotus or easy pose. Put the hands on the knees in gyan mudra. Let the eyes be nearly closed. Break the inhale into 10 equal parts or "sniffs." With each part of the inhale move the hands mechanically (in small jerks) one-tenth of the way toward the forehead. The palms face up and all the fingers are straight during the inhale. At the tenth inhale the palms are on the forehead with the fingers pointing up. As you exhale join the fingertips of the two hands and let the hands down slowly. Separate the hands at the level of the navel point and return them to gyan mudra in the original position. On each inhale mentally vibrate the mantra **Wahe**. On the exhale vibrate **Guru**. Continue for 3 to 11 minutes.

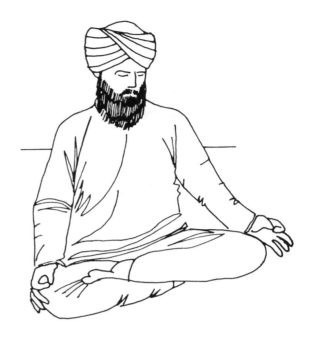

COMMENTS:

This kriya builds the nervous system so nothing bothers you. It stimulates the pituitary to secrete and gives you an expanded intuitive sense. It makes the mind clear and decisive. If the aura and nerves lack strength it is difficult to act on ideals you have. This kriya helps you directly direct yourself.

Begin the practice with only a few minutes. Then build slowly up to 11 minutes.

GURU RAM DAS:
RHYTHMIC HARMONY
FOR HAPPINESS

Sit in a peaceful meditative pose. Keep the eyes one-sixteenth open. Men take the left hand and form Shuni mudra with the thumb and middle finger. With the right hand, join the thumb to the tip of the ring finger (for women, the mudras are reversed). Rest the hands on the knees. Chant in a soft monotone:

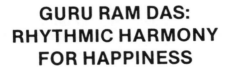

Guru Guru Wahe Guru
Guru Ram Das Guru

Each repetition takes about 8 to 10 seconds. Continue for 11 to 31 minutes.

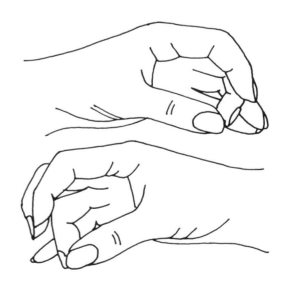

COMMENTS:

The Siri Singh Sahib said when he taught this that it "is to bring to the self a meditative peace. This is a *maithuna*. It's so vibratory even your lips, your upper palate, your tongue, your entire surroundings feel a vibratory effect. It's my personal mantra. It was given to me by Guru Ram Das in his astral self, not when I was challenged, but when Guru Ram Das was challenged. The beauty of this mantra is that it was tested. When our lives were in danger I said, 'Folks, keep on chanting this. We'll always be protected.' It's the same today. It always will be through every moment of life. It is called ecstasy of consciousness. The impossible becomes pure, simple, truthfully possible because you have the given values and you have given yourself, soul and spirit, to those given values righteously. It is then that God manifests everything. And that's why we chant in this mudra this simple mantra."

BRAHM MUDRA MEDITATION

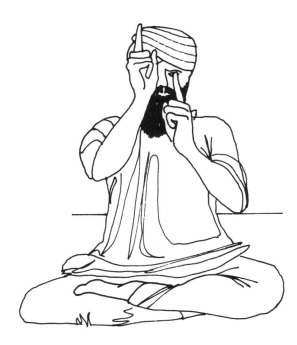

Sit with the spine straight. Make fists of both hands. The thumb should be on the outside of the fist with Jupiter fingers pointing straight up. Hold the two hands so that they face each other. The left hand is lower, the left Jupiter fingertip being exactly even with the lowest knuckle of the right thumb. The two hands are like conches pointing to God. The eyes are open, looking straight and directly at and through the space of the hands. Hold the hands about 1 to 1½ feet from the face. Keep the neck straight. Mentally meditate on **Ad Guray Nameh, Jugad Guray Nameh, Sat Guray Nameh, Siri Guru Devay Nameh**. After 11 minutes close the eyes and, holding the position, chant aloud the mantra in a monotone and in a simple, moderate rhythm.

COMMENTS:

This mudra symbolizes yin and yang pointing towards God. It is a mudra of immediate spirit and protection. All previous incarnations, the present, and the future shall be directed towards righteousness. This mudra changes the metabolism of the mind and develops a "funny mandala" called "Brahm Mandala."

Brahm mudra is good for outrageous behavior, tremendous depression, and inconsistency in character. It creates happiness on the spot where there is unhappiness.

THE 3HO FOUNDATION

The Healthy, Happy, Holy Organization, 3HO Foundation, is dedicated to serving God and humanity. It is basically a teacher-training institution which uses Kundalini yoga as a technique for raising consciousness and expanding awareness. 3HO International Headquarters is located in Los Angeles, California.

The Siri Singh Sahib, master of Kundalini and Tantric yogas, teaches a superb lecture-meditation series at the headquarters from September through May. He also travels throughout the world conducting courses in meditation and Tantric yoga.

If you would like to be on the mailing list to receive his current teaching itinerary, write to

3HO Foundation
International Headquarters
House of Guru Ram Das
1620 Preuss Road
Los Angeles, CA 90035

THE KUNDALINI RESEARCH INSTITUTE

K.R.I., the Kundalini Research Institute, was established to verify, scientifically, the effects of practicing Kundalini yoga, to publish the results of their investigations, and to make the teachings of the Siri Singh Sahib available to everybody. This manual is one of many publications published by the institute. If you are interested in receiving a list of current materials, write us at

Kundalini Research Institute
c/o G.T. International
1800 S. Robertson Blvd.
Suite 182
Los Angeles, CA 90035
(213) 551-0484

We welcome your questions, comments and suggestions.

THE JOURNEY

Yogi Bhajan, PhD

"This world and our journey in life is actually very clear.
Every aspect of it is organized and creative.
We are supposed to live with each other in love,
Work as a worship,
And follow the path of righteousness
to propel our consciousness across the cycle of time."

PART I

MORNING SADHANA FOR THE AQUARIAN AGE

Throughout the years Yogi Bhajan has periodically adjusted the content of our morning sadhana. He gave us the following sequence of mantras on June 21, 1992, with instructions to continue chanting them in this order for 21 years. So, until the year 2013, we are set with the best sadhana tools possible. There is no time gap or pause between the different mantra sections. Total time is 62 minutes.

1. Ek Ong Kar Sat Nam Siri Wahe Guru

(7 minutes)

"One Creator created this Creation. Truth is His Name. Great beyond description is His infinite wisdom."

The cornerstone of morning sadhana is *"Long Ek Ong Kar's."* This Ashtang Mantra is sometimes called "Morning Call." *(Please refer to pages 37-38 for the technology on how to chant this mantra and for a more detailed explanation of its meaning and effects.)* It is essential that you:

- Sit with a straight spine.
- Apply neck lock (Jalander Bandh) by pulling the chin straight back.

Inhale deeply and chant **EK ONG KAAR**.

Inhale deeply again and chant **SAT Naaam** until you're almost out of breath, then REACH for the **S'ree**, which is brief.

Then, inhale 1/2 Breath and chant **WAH-HAY GU'ROO**

Inhale deeply again to repeat the cycle.

"Long Ek Ong Kar's" are chanted without musical accompaniment, whereas the six mantras that follow may be chanted using various melodies with or without instrumental accompaniment. (Musicians take note: instruments are for background to accompany and support the voice. Also, please be sure to preserve the original rhythm of the mantra by keeping the length of the syllables intact.)

2. Waah Yantee, Kar Yantee (7 minutes)

Waah Yantee, Kar Yantee
Jag Doot Patee, Aadak It Waahaa
Brahmaadeh Traysha Guru
It Waahe Guru

Great Macroself, Creative Self.
All that is creative through time.
All that is the Great One. Three aspects of God:
Brahma, Vishnu, Mahesh (Shiva).
That is Wahe Guru.

3. The Mool Mantra (7 minutes)

The Mool (Root) Mantra lets you experience the depth and conciousness of your soul.

a) IMPORTANT: Leave a slight "space" (not a breath) between *ajoonee* and *saibhang.* Do not run the words together.

b) Emphasize and slightly extend the "ch" sound at the end of the word *sach.* This adds power.

Ek Ong Kaar	One Creator, Creation
Sat Naam	Truth Identified (Named)
Kartaa Purakh	Doer of Everything
Nirbhao	Fearless
Nirvair	Revengeless
Akaal Moorat	Undying
Ajoonee	Unborn
Saibhang	Self-illumined, self-existent
Gur Prasaad	Guru's grace (gift)
Jap!	REPEAT (Chant)
Aad Sach	True in the beginning
Jugaad Sach	True throughout the Ages
Hai Bhee Sach	True even now
Naanak Hosee Bhee Sach	
	Nanak says Truth shall ever be

This mantra gives you the capacity to retain rulership. There are 108 elements in the universe, and 108 letters in this mantra (in the original Gurmukhi script—counting all vowels as letters).

4. Sat Siri, Siri Akal (7 minutes)
"The Mantra for the Aquarian Age."

Sat Siri	Great Truth
Siri Akaal	Great Undying
Siri Akaal	Great Undying
Maha Akaal	Great Deathless
Maha Akaal	Great Deathless
Sat Naam	Truth is His Name
Akaal Moorat	Deathless Image of God
Wahe Guru	Great beyond description is His Wisdom

5. Rakhe Rakhan Har (7 minutes)
This is a sound current of protection against all negative forces which move against one's walk on the path of destiny, both inner and outer. It cuts like a sword through every opposing vibration, thought, word, and action.

It is part of the evening prayer of the Sikhs (Rehiras). Rakhe Rakhan Har was composed by Guru Arjan Dev, the Fifth Guru.

Rakhay rakhanahaar aap ubaaria-an
Gur kee pairee paa-ay kaaj savaari-an
Hoaa aap day-aal manaho na visaari-an
Saadh janaa kai sang bhavajal taari-an
Saakat nindak dusht khin maa-eh bidaari-an
Tis saahib kee tayk Naanak manai maa-eh
Jis simrat sukh ho-ay sagalay dookh jaa-eh

(The following translation was given by Yogi Bhajan on June 15, 1986, in St. Louis, Missouri.)

*Thou who savest, save us all and take us across,
Uplifting and giving the excellence.
You gave us the touch of the lotus feet of the
    Guru, and all our jobs are done.
You have become merciful, kind, and
    compassionate; and so our mind does
    not forget Thee.*

*In the company of the holy beings you take us
    from misfortune and calamities, scandals,
    and disrepute.
Godless, slandeorus enemies—you finish them in
    timelessness.
That great Lord is my anchor.
Nanak, keep Him firm in your mind.
By meditating and repeating his Name,
All happiness comes and all sorrows and
    pain go away.*

6. Wahe Guru Wahe Jio (22 minutes)
To be most effective, chant this mantra sitting in Vir Asan, as follows: Sit on your left heel, with the right knee against the chest, and the hands in prayer pose. Eyes are focused at the tip of the nose.

Wahe Guru Wahe Guru Wahe Guru Wahe Jeeo

Wahe Guru is a mantra of ecstasy. There is no real translation for it, though we could say, *"Wow, God is great!"*, or *"Indescribably great is His Infinite, Ultimate Wisdom."* *Jeeo* is an affectionate but still respectful variation of the word *Jee* which means soul.

7. Guru Ram Das Chant (5 minutes)
Guru Guru Wahe Guru Guru Raam Das Guru

These syllables are in praise of the consciousness of Guru Ram Das (the Fourth Sikh Guru) and invoke his spiritual light, guidance, and protective grace.

THE SEVEN STEPS TO HAPPINESS

Yogi Bhajan, PhD

"Commitment leads to Character

Character leads to Dignity

Dignity leads to Divinity

Divinity leads to Grace

Grace leads to the power to Sacrifice

The Power to Sacrifice leads to Happiness"

NOTES

THE 3HO FOUNDATION

The Healthy, Happy, Holy Organization, 3HO Foundation, is dedicated to serving God and humanity. It is basically a teacher-training institution which uses Kundalini Yoga as a technique for raising consciousness and expanding awareness. 3HO International Headquarters is located in Los Angeles, California.

Yogi Bhajan, Master of Kundalini and Yoga and Mahan Tantric of White Tantric Yoga, teaches around the world with regularly scheduled courses in Los Angeles, CA, and Espanola, NM.

If you would like to be on the mailing list to receive course and event information, please write to:

3HO Foundation
P.O. Box 351149
Los Angeles, CA 90035

THE KUNDALINI RESEARCH INSTITUTE

K.R.I., the Kundalini Research Institute, was created to establish and preserve the legacy of the Teachings of Yogi Bhajan. It facilitates the organization and publication of Kundalini Yoga and meditation technologies into books, manuals, video and audio tapes, and electronic media. KRI also licenses KRI Teacher Training courses.

This manual is one of many products available. To receive a listing of publications, please contact:

Ancient Healing Ways Catalog
Tel 800-359-2940 inside the US
Tel 505-747-2860 outside the US
Fax 505-747-2868

For information on Kundalini Yoga classes and teachers, please contact:
International Kundalini Yoga Teachers Association:
Tel 505-753-0423
Internet: www.yogibhajan.com